Envisioning a Transformed Clinical Trials Enterprise for 2030

PROCEEDINGS OF A WORKSHOP

Theresa Wizemann, Amanda Wagner Gee, and Carolyn Shore,
Rapporteurs

Forum on Drug Discovery, Development, and Translation

Board on Health Sciences Policy

Health and Medicine Division

The National Academies of
SCIENCES · ENGINEERING · MEDICINE

THE NATIONAL ACADEMIES PRESS
Washington, DC
www.nap.edu

THE NATIONAL ACADEMIES PRESS   500 Fifth Street, NW   Washington, DC 20001

This activity was supported by contracts between the National Academy of Sciences and Amgen Inc.; Association of American Medical Colleges; AstraZeneca; Biogen; Biomedical Advanced Research and Development Authority; Burroughs Wellcome Fund (Contract No. 1021334); Critical Path Institute; Eli Lilly and Company (Contract No. 4900709231); FasterCures, Milken Institute; Foundation for the National Institutes of Health; Friends of Cancer Research; Johnson & Johnson; Medable; Merck & Co., Inc. (Contract No. MRLCPO-21-138769); National Institutes of Health (Contract No. HHSN263201800029I; Task Order No. HHSN26300007): National Cancer Institute, National Institute of Allergy and Infectious Diseases, National Institute of Mental Health, National Institute of Neurological Disorders and Stroke, Office of Science Policy; *New England Journal of Medicine*; Sanofi (Contract No. 65873711); Takeda Pharmaceuticals; U.S. Food and Drug Administration (Grant No. 1R13FD007302-01). Any opinions, findings, conclusions, or recommendations expressed in this publication do not necessarily reflect the views of any organization or agency that provided support for the project.

International Standard Book Number-13: 978-0-309-26928-5
International Standard Book Number-10: 0-309-26928-8
Digital Object Identifier: https://doi.org/10.17226/26349

Additional copies of this publication are available from the National Academies Press, 500 Fifth Street, NW, Keck 360, Washington, DC 20001; (800) 624-6242 or (202) 334-3313; http://www.nap.edu.

Copyright 2022 by the National Academy of Sciences. All rights reserved.

Printed in the United States of America

Suggested citation: National Academies of Sciences, Engineering, and Medicine. 2022. *Envisioning a transformed clinical trials enterprise for 2030: Proceedings of a workshop*. Washington, DC: The National Academies Press. https://doi.org/10.17226/26349.

The National Academies of
SCIENCES · ENGINEERING · MEDICINE

The **National Academy of Sciences** was established in 1863 by an Act of Congress, signed by President Lincoln, as a private, nongovernmental institution to advise the nation on issues related to science and technology. Members are elected by their peers for outstanding contributions to research. Dr. Marcia McNutt is president.

The **National Academy of Engineering** was established in 1964 under the charter of the National Academy of Sciences to bring the practices of engineering to advising the nation. Members are elected by their peers for extraordinary contributions to engineering. Dr. John L. Anderson is president.

The **National Academy of Medicine** (formerly the Institute of Medicine) was established in 1970 under the charter of the National Academy of Sciences to advise the nation on medical and health issues. Members are elected by their peers for distinguished contributions to medicine and health. Dr. Victor J. Dzau is president.

The three Academies work together as the **National Academies of Sciences, Engineering, and Medicine** to provide independent, objective analysis and advice to the nation and conduct other activities to solve complex problems and inform public policy decisions. The National Academies also encourage education and research, recognize outstanding contributions to knowledge, and increase public understanding in matters of science, engineering, and medicine.

Learn more about the National Academies of Sciences, Engineering, and Medicine at **www.nationalacademies.org**.

The National Academies of
SCIENCES • ENGINEERING • MEDICINE

Consensus Study Reports published by the National Academies of Sciences, Engineering, and Medicine document the evidence-based consensus on the study's statement of task by an authoring committee of experts. Reports typically include findings, conclusions, and recommendations based on information gathered by the committee and the committee's deliberations. Each report has been subjected to a rigorous and independent peer-review process and it represents the position of the National Academies on the statement of task.

Proceedings published by the National Academies of Sciences, Engineering, and Medicine chronicle the presentations and discussions at a workshop, symposium, or other event convened by the National Academies. The statements and opinions contained in proceedings are those of the participants and are not endorsed by other participants, the planning committee, or the National Academies.

For information about other products and activities of the National Academies, please visit www.nationalacademies.org/about/whatwedo.

ENVISIONING A TRANSFORMED CLINICAL TRIALS ENTERPRISE FOR 2030[1]

STEVEN GALSON (*Co-Chair*), Amgen Inc.
ESTHER KROFAH (*Co-Chair*), FasterCures, Milken Institute
AMY ABERNETHY, Verily Life Sciences
ANITA ALLEN, University of Pennsylvania Carey School of Law
CHRISTOPHER AUSTIN, Flagship Pioneering
HOWARD BURRIS, Sarah Cannon
LUTHER CLARK, Merck & Co., Inc.
GISELLE CORBIE-SMITH, University of North Carolina School of Medicine
M. KHAIR ELZARRAD, Center for Drug Evaluation and Safety, U.S. Food and Drug Administration
JENNIFER GOLDSACK, Digital Medicine Society
RICHARD MOSCICKI, PhRMA
AMY PATTERSON, National Heart, Lung, and Blood Institute, National Institutes of Health
JOSEPH SCHEEREN, Retired
ANANTHA SHEKHAR, University of Pittsburgh
PAMELA TENAERTS, Medable Inc.
CHRISTOPHER YOO, Systems Oncology

Health and Medicine Division Staff

CAROLYN K. SHORE, Director, Forum on Drug Discovery, Development, and Translation
AMANDA WAGNER GEE, Program Officer
JULIE LIAO, Program Officer
ANDREW MARCH, Associate Program Officer
MELVIN JOPPY, Senior Program Assistant
ANDREW M. POPE, Senior Director, Board on Health Sciences Policy

Consultant

THERESA WIZEMANN, Science Writer

---

[1] The National Academies of Sciences, Engineering, and Medicine's planning committees are solely responsible for organizing the workshop, identifying topics, and choosing speakers. The responsibility for the published Proceedings of a Workshop rests with the workshop rapporteurs and the institution.

FORUM ON DRUG DISCOVERY, DEVELOPMENT, AND TRANSLATION[1]

ROBERT M. CALIFF (*Co-Chair*), Duke University and Verily Life Sciences and Google Health
GREGORY SIMON (*Co-Chair*), Kaiser Permanente Washington Health Research Institute and University of Washington
CHRISTOPHER P. AUSTIN, Flagship Pioneering
LINDA BRADY, National Institute of Mental Health, National Institutes of Health
JOHN BUSE, University of North Carolina School of Medicine
BARRY S. COLLER, The Rockefeller University
THOMAS CURRAN, Children's Mercy, Kansas City
RICHARD DAVEY, National Institute of Allergy and Infectious Diseases, National Institutes of Health
KATHERINE DAWSON, Biogen
JAMES H. DOROSHOW, National Cancer Institute, National Institutes of Health
JEFFREY M. DRAZEN, *New England Journal of Medicine*
STEVEN K. GALSON, Amgen Inc.
CARLOS O. GARNER, Eli Lilly and Company
JULIE L. GERBERDING, Merck & Co., Inc.
DEBORAH HUNG, Harvard Medical School
LYRIC JORGENSON, Office of Science Policy, National Institutes of Health
ESTHER KROFAH, FasterCures, Milken Institute
LISA M. LaVANGE, University of North Carolina
LEANNE MADRE, Clinical Trials Transformation Initiative
ROSS McKINNEY, JR., Association of American Medical Colleges
JOSEPH P. MENETSKI, Foundation for the National Institutes of Health
ARTI RAI, Duke University School of Law
MARK ROGGE, Retired
KLAUS ROMERO, Critical Path Institute
KELLY ROSE, Burroughs Wellcome Fund
SUSAN SCHAEFFER, Patients' Academy for Research Advocacy
JOSEPH SCHEEREN, Retired
ANANTHA SHEKHAR, University of Pittsburgh
JAY SIEGEL, Retired
ELLEN V. SIGAL, Friends of Cancer Research

---

[1] The National Academies of Sciences, Engineering, and Medicine's forums and roundtables do not issue, review, or approve individual documents. The responsibility for the published Proceedings of a Workshop rests with the workshop rapporteurs and the institution.

LANA R. SKIRBOLL, Sanofi
AMIR TAMIZ, National Institute of Neurological Disorders and Stroke, National Institutes of Health
ANN TAYLOR, AstraZeneca
PAMELA TENAERTS, Medable Inc.
JOANNE WALDSTREICHER, Johnson & Johnson
ROBERT WALKER, Biomedical Advanced Research and Development Authority
JONATHAN WATANABE, University of California, Irvine, School of Pharmacy and Pharmaceutical Sciences
ALASTAIR WOOD, Vanderbilt University
JANET WOODCOCK, U.S. Food and Drug Administration

Forum Staff

CAROLYN K. SHORE, Forum Director
AMANDA WAGNER GEE, Program Officer
ANDREW MARCH, Associate Program Officer
MELVIN JOPPY, Senior Program Assistant
ANDREW M. POPE, Senior Director, Board on Health Sciences Policy

Reviewers

This Proceedings of a Workshop was reviewed in draft form by individuals chosen for their diverse perspectives and technical expertise. The purpose of this independent review is to provide candid and critical comments that will assist the National Academies of Sciences, Engineering, and Medicine in making each published proceedings as sound as possible and to ensure that it meets the institutional standards for quality, objectivity, evidence, and responsiveness to the charge. The review comments and draft manuscript remain confidential to protect the integrity of the process.

We thank the following individuals for their review of this proceedings:

BARBARA BIERER, Harvard Medical School
BARRY COLLER, The Rockefeller University
M. KHAIR ELZARRAD, U.S. Food and Drug Administration
JOHN ORLOFF, Alexion (Retired)

Although the reviewers listed above provided many constructive comments and suggestions, they were not asked to endorse the content of the proceedings nor did they see the final draft before its release. The review of this proceedings was overseen by **ELI ADASHI,** Brown University. He was responsible for making certain that an independent examination of this proceedings was carried out in accordance with standards of the National Academies and that all review comments were carefully considered. Responsibility for the final content rests entirely with the rapporteurs and the National Academies.

Acknowledgments

Support from the sponsors of the Forum on Drug Discovery, Development, and Translation is crucial to support this and other work of the National Academies.

The National Academies staff wish to express their gratitude to the speakers whose presentations helped inform workshop discussions on the state of drug research and development for adults across the older age span; to the members of the planning committee for their work in developing the workshop agenda and shaping the discussions; and to National Academies staff without whom this workshop and the accounting thereof would not have been possible: Christie Bell, Robert Day, Sadaf Faraz, Eeshan Khandekar, Devona Overton, Esther Pak, Marguerite Romatelli, Bettina Seliber, Lauren Shern, and Taryn Young.

Contents

ACRONYMS AND ABBREVIATIONS   xvii

1   INTRODUCTION   1
     Organization of the Workshop and Proceedings, 3

2   DEFINING THE VISION   5
     Envisioning a More Person-Centered and Inclusive Clinical
        Trials Enterprise, 6
     Envisioning an Optimized Clinical Trials Enterprise Through
        the Use of Technologies, 9
     Envisioning a More Resilient, Sustainable, and Transparent
        Clinical Trials Enterprise, 13

3   ENHANCING OUTCOMES IN A MORE PERSON-CENTERED
     AND INCLUSIVE CLINICAL TRIALS ENTERPRISE   19
     The Road to 2030: Perspectives from the Field, 20
     The Road to 2030: Visions of What Is Possible, 24
     Reflections on Achieving Person-Centered and Inclusive Trials, 32

4   PRACTICAL APPLICATIONS FOR TECHNOLOGY TO
     ENHANCE THE CLINICAL TRIALS ENTERPRISE   35
     The Road to 2030: Perspectives from the Field, 36
     The Road to 2030: Visions of What Is Possible, 40

Reflections on Realizing the Potential of Technology in Clinical
     Trials, 45

5 BUILDING A MORE RESILIENT, SUSTAINABLE, AND
  TRANSPARENT CLINICAL TRIALS ENTERPRISE   49
  The Road to 2030: Perspectives from the Field, 50
  The Road to 2030: Visions of What Is Possible, 57
  Reflections on Resilience, Sustainability, and Transparency of
     the Clinical Trials Enterprise, 66

6 OPPORTUNITIES FOR TRANSFORMATION   69
  Opportunities to Transform the Clinical Trials Enterprise, 70
  Innovating for 2030 Now, 73
  Taking the Lessons from the COVID-19 Pandemic Response
     Forward, 75
  Closing Remarks, 77

REFERENCES   79

APPENDIXES

A *HEALTH AFFAIRS* BLOG POSTS   81
B SPEAKER AND MODERATOR BIOGRAPHIES   83
C WORKSHOP AGENDAS   107

Boxes and Figures

BOXES

1-1 Workshop Statement of Task, 2

5-1 Lessons from RECOVERY, 53

FIGURES

2-1 One sponsor's qualitative impression of the adoption and impact of remote approaches on the conduct of clinical trials during a pandemic, 15

5-1 Basic protocol design for the first phase of the RECOVERY trial, 51
5-2 Complexity of community, 61

Acronyms and Abbreviations

AAMC	Association of American Medical Colleges
ACTIV	Accelerating COVID-19 Therapeutic Interventions and Vaccines (NIH)
CBER	Center for Biologics Evaluation and Research (FDA)
CDER	Center for Drug Evaluation and Research (FDA)
CEAL	Community Engagement Alliance (NIH)
CEO	chief executive officer
CMS	Centers for Medicare & Medicaid Services
CoVPN	COVID-19 Prevention Network
CTTI	Clinical Trials Transformation Initiative
EHR	electronic health record
FDA	U.S. Food and Drug Administration
FDASIA	U.S. Food and Drug Administration Safety and Innovation Act
GDPR	General Data Protection Regulation
HBCU	Historically Black College and University
HEAL	Healthy Eating Active Living
HRSA	Health Resources and Services Administration

IRB	institutional review board
NCATS	National Center for Advancing Translational Sciences
NHS	National Health Service (United Kingdom)
NIH	National Institutes of Health (United States)
NIMHD	National Institute on Minority Health and Health Disparities
OMHHE	Office of Minority Health and Health Equity
PCORI	Patient-Centered Outcomes Research Institute
PDUFA	Prescription Drug User Fee Act
R&D	research and development
RECOVERY	Randomized Evaluation of COVID-19 Therapy Trials

1

Introduction[1]

The conduct and design of clinical trials has changed considerably over the past decade since the 2011 Institute of Medicine workshop Envisioning a Transformed Clinical Trials Enterprise in the United States: Establishing an Agenda for 2020 (IOM, 2012). The evolution of health care is expanding the possibilities for integration of clinical research into the continuum of clinical care; new approaches are enabling the collection of data in real-world settings; and new modalities, such as digital health technologies[2] and artificial intelligence applications, are being leveraged to overcome challenges and advance clinical research. At the same time, the clinical research enterprise is strained by rising costs, varying global regulatory and economic landscapes, increasing complexity of clinical trials, barriers to recruitment and retention of research participants, and a clinical research workforce that is under tremendous demands.

---

[1] This workshop was organized by an independent planning committee whose role was limited to identification of topics and speakers. This Proceedings of a Workshop was prepared by the rapporteurs as a factual summary of the presentations and discussions that took place at the workshop. Statements, recommendations, and opinions expressed are those of individual presenters and participants and are not endorsed or verified by the National Academies of Sciences, Engineering, and Medicine, and they should not be construed as reflecting any group consensus.

[2] Defined as ranging "from hardware—such as wearable devices and sensors—to software, such as mobile phone apps that enable consumers to monitor their own health and participate in studies; telemedicine platforms to connect patients with clinical providers; and artificial intelligence to support clinical decision making" (NASEM, 2020, p. 1).

> **BOX 1-1**
> **Workshop Statement of Task**
>
> A planning committee of the National Academies of Sciences, Engineering, and Medicine will plan and conduct a virtual, four-part public workshop designed to consider a transformed clinical trials enterprise for 2030, featuring invited presentations and discussions on:
>
> - Lessons learned from progress and setbacks over the past 10 years.
> - How an envisioned 2030 clinical trials enterprise might differ from the current system.
> - The following core themes in framing a 2030 agenda:
>   - Diversity and inclusion of clinical trial participants
>   - Convergence of clinical research and clinical practice
>   - Clinical trial data sharing
>   - Incorporation of new technologies into drug research and development
>   - Workforce and career development
>   - Public engagement and partnership
>   - Regulatory environment
>   - Cultural and financial incentives
> - Key priority challenges and opportunities when it comes to the 2030 clinical trials enterprise.
> - Practical short- and long-term goals for improving the efficiency, effectiveness, person-centeredness, inclusivity, and integration with health care of the clinical trials enterprise.

Looking ahead to 2030, the Forum on Drug Discovery, Development, and Translation of the National Academies of Sciences, Engineering, and Medicine (the National Academies) convened a public workshop for stakeholders from across the drug research and development (R&D) life cycle to reflect on the lessons learned over the past 10 years and consider opportunities for the future. The agenda for the workshop was developed by an independent planning committee to address the established task (see Box 1-1).[3] Specifically, the workshop was designed to consider goals and priority action items that could advance the vision of a 2030 clinical trials enterprise that is more efficient, effective, person-centered, inclusive, and integrated into the health care delivery system so that outcomes and experiences for all stakeholders are improved. The workshop was co-chaired by Esther Krofah, executive director at FasterCures, a center of the Milken Institute, and Steven Galson, senior vice president of Research and Development at Amgen Inc.

---

[3] The agendas for the four parts of the workshop can be found in Appendix C.

INTRODUCTION   3

Originally intended to be held in person in Washington, DC, over the course of 1.5 days, the workshop was redesigned as a four-part virtual event spanning 5 months due to the COVID-19 pandemic and the need to hold the workshop virtually. At the time of the first meeting in January 2021, more than 25 million people in the United States had been infected with COVID-19, and more than 400,000 had died as a result.[4] "We have witnessed a tremendous response from the medical research community in accelerating the development of therapeutics and vaccines," said Krofah. In January 2021, two vaccines had already shown sufficient evidence of safety and efficacy in clinical trials to be authorized for emergency use by the U.S. Food and Drug Administration (FDA). At the same time, however, the pandemic resulted in the disruption of new and existing clinical trials for a range of diseases. "It's clear that we have an urgent need, now more than ever, to advance a clinical trials enterprise that is more efficient, effective, person-centered, inclusive, and integrated into the health delivery system," Krofah said.

ORGANIZATION OF THE WORKSHOP AND PROCEEDINGS

This Proceedings of a Workshop summarizes the presentations and discussions that took place during the four-part virtual public workshop held on January 26, February 9, March 24, and May 11, 2021.[5] All four parts of the workshop, including interactive breakout group discussions, were facilitated remotely via Zoom and webcast live. Participants were also able to submit comments and questions throughout the workshop via the webcast comment window or within a dedicated Slack workspace.

Chapter 2 provides an overview of some changes in communities and clinical research as a result of the COVID-19 pandemic, lessons learned from the positive and negative effects of those changes, and ways in which an envisioned 2030 clinical trials enterprise could differ from the current system. It introduces some of the key challenges and opportunities for achieving that vision. Chapter 3 summarizes workshop discussions focused on achievable goals to enhance person-centeredness and inclusivity throughout the clinical trials enterprise and ways to improve public engagement and partnership. Chapter 4 covers discussions on how the thoughtful and deliberate use of new technologies could enhance the clinical trials enterprise. Chapter 5 recaps the workshop discussions in

---

[4] This information is from the Johns Hopkins University Coronavirus Resource Center. For more information and updated counts, see https://coronavirus.jhu.edu/us-map (accessed September 9, 2021).

[5] Archived webcast videos and additional meeting materials are available on the National Academies website. See https://www.nationalacademies.org/our-work/envisioning-a-transformed-clinical-trials-enterprise-for-2030-a-workshop (accessed July 19, 2021).

which participants considered approaches to building a more resilient, sustainable, and transparent clinical trials enterprise, including the integration of clinical research and clinical practice. Throughout Chapters 3, 4, and 5, many individual workshop speakers and participants drew examples from their experiences and observations during the COVID-19 pandemic, and discussed the potential for some of those lessons learned to inform an envisioned transformation of the clinical trials enterprise.

Over the course of the workshop, three current and former FDA officials shared their personal perspectives on the state of the clinical trials enterprise, changes made as a result of the COVID-19 pandemic, examples of positive changes made that potentially could be continued post-pandemic, and what it may take to realize the 2030 vision. These discussions are summarized in Chapter 6, which also includes closing remarks from the workshop co-chairs. A series of *Health Affairs* blog posts were written by select workshop speakers to complement the workshop discussions (see Appendix A).[6] Participants were encouraged to share their insights and observations about the workshop on Twitter using the hashtags #ClinicalTrials2030 and #DrugForum.

---

[6] See https://www.healthaffairs.org/topic/ss170 (accessed July 1, 2021).

2

Defining the Vision

> **Highlights of Key Points Made by Individual Speakers**
> - Distrust of the biomedical research and health care systems persists. (King)
> - Building trust with Black communities involves making their health a priority and being transparent about the process and the products of medical research. (King)
> - Digital health technologies can enable research to be conducted at the scale needed for studies to be representative, reliable, and adequately powered to produce meaningful data. (Califf)
> - The quality of electronic health record data and claims data is improving, and standards, common data models, and the automated curation methods that are being developed and deployed can help support the advancement of a learning health system. (Califf)
> - The interests of the sponsors, patients, and societies are not necessarily in conflict. A more patient- and society-focused clinical research enterprise can also be more efficient and productive for industry trial sponsors. (Levy)
> - Improving industry efficiency can help reduce the burden of trial participation for patients and increase the volume of data available to support societies in evidence-based, health-related decision making. (Levy)

To open the workshop, three speakers shared their personal perspectives on key focus areas of the series: person-centeredness and inclusivity in clinical trials; the role of digital technology in conducting clinical trials; and resilience, sustainability, and transparency of the clinical trials enterprise. Terris King, former director of the Office of Minority Health at the Centers for Medicare & Medicaid Services (CMS), shared his vision for building a more person-centered and inclusive clinical trials enterprise by 2030. Robert Califf, head of Clinical Strategy and Policy at Verily Life Sciences and Google Health, reflected on the use of existing and emerging technologies for achieving the aspirations for a transformed 2030 clinical trials enterprise. Elliott Levy, senior vice president for R&D Strategy and Operation at Amgen Inc., shared his vision for a future of clinical research that could better meet the needs of patients and society. Each talk was followed by a facilitated breakout group discussion.

ENVISIONING A MORE PERSON-CENTERED AND INCLUSIVE CLINICAL TRIALS ENTERPRISE

A Perspective on Person-Centeredness and Inclusivity: Moving Forward Together

King's community has experienced high rates of COVID-19 cases during the pandemic. He described his work participating in focus groups for Johns Hopkins University and the Robert Wood Johnson Foundation, and arranging for conversations between several pharmaceutical companies and his congregation to discuss vaccination and to address issues with misinformation. Through these activities, King heard that distrust of the biomedical research and health care systems persists. He told workshop participants that "many African Americans … would rather die than take a vaccine that many of you would offer." He shared the perspective that many from his community believe that others only care about the health of Black communities now given the COVID-19 pandemic because they realize everyone's health is interconnected. The sense of many Black communities around the country, King said, is that "if entities talking to us would talk about more than vaccine hesitancy, if health care institutions would also talk about the health issues and concerns that we had before COVID ever came, we might trust that they're actually meaning us good for when this is over, and we might actually listen to them in terms of taking a vaccine."

Long before the pandemic, the promise of precision medicine was that treatment of disease could be tailored to individuals based on genetic and other factors. At the time, King said, the need for greater participation by African Americans and other underrepresented minorities in clinical trials was acknowledged. Yet, minority populations are still underrepresented in clinical trials, hindering the development and application of precision medicine treatments that could benefit them. "We [Black communities and clinical trialists] need each other in terms of trials," King said. "We need each other in terms of participation. We need each other to move forward." African Americans suffer from high rates of diabetes, hypertension, and obesity (NCHS, 2021), and are more likely to die from COVID-19 than white Americans (CDC, 2021). Many researchers, clinicians, and policy experts have suggested that the disparity in COVID-19 mortality rates might be associated with social determinants of health and/or underlying comorbidities, such as diabetes, but the true reason is still unknown. Understanding and addressing the health concerns of African Americans has not been a priority for research, King noted.

Building trust with Black communities involves making the health of African Americans a priority and being transparent about the process and the products of medical research. King said the clinical trials enterprise is using "the wrong message and the wrong messengers" when trying to engage minority populations in clinical trials. What is needed, he continued, is a person-centered model of community-based participatory research that reaches African Americans in the spaces where they gather to share their faith and their fears and where trusted relationships are built. These spaces include not just churches, but also community sanctuaries such as beauty salons and barbershops. Trusted community members and pastors in these spaces can work with researchers and the pharmaceutical industry to build programs that convey, with complete transparency, the benefit of the pharmaceutical products for the community.

King emphasized the need to invest in the community, and provide stipends to the trusted community members to enable them to educate and engage others in the research process. "What we discovered from COVID is we're connected. Let's use this process to connect and build processes that work for both parties," he said, adding that both parties must humble themselves so they can learn from each other. He noted that this approach to engaging the community is not new and has been successful in other health settings (e.g., Project Dulce for improving diabetes care in underrepresented populations).[1] In conclusion, King said, "Let's work together and build a vision for 2030 to save the least, the lost, and those who lack support."

---

[1] For more information, see https://www.scripps.org/services/metabolic-conditions/diabetes/diabetes-professional-training (accessed August 3, 2021).

Enhancing Outcomes in a More Person-Centered and Inclusive Clinical Trials Enterprise: Breakout Discussion Highlights

A summary of the points made by individual breakout group participants was provided in plenary session by Natalie Rotelli of Eli Lilly and Company, Mark Unruh of The University of New Mexico, Jonathan Watanabe of the University of California, Irvine, and Jeanne Regnante of the LUNGevity Foundation on behalf of four breakout groups. The following topics were highlighted by breakout group participants as being of interest for further discussion in the subsequent workshop meetings (see Chapter 3). This section is the rapporteurs' summary of the breakout group reports by Rotelli, Unruh, Watanabe, and Regnante, and should not be construed as reflecting agreement among any group. All suggestions and proposals are reported for discussion purposes only.

Improving Representation and Relevance

The results of a clinical trial should be relevant to trial participants and to the broader patient population. Breakout discussants observed that only a small subset of the general population participates in clinical trials, which compounds the challenges of enrolling a diverse and representative trial population. Participants discussed how elements of study design could create barriers to participation for minorities (e.g., inclusion and exclusion criteria, convenience of site locations, or appointment hours) and how new approaches to participation that leverage digital health technologies might increase access to clinical trial participation. The need for metrics to demonstrate progress toward the goal of improving representation and relevance was raised by discussants, and it was noted that measures of success should be driven by what is meaningful to communities.

Engaging and Preparing a More Diverse Clinical Research Workforce

Representation applies not only to trial participants, but also to those designing and conducting the trials. Breakout discussants suggested that the clinical trials workforce should reflect the community it serves. Engaging investigators beyond those affiliated with traditional academic research institutions was discussed as one way to broaden diverse representation among both investigators and participants, and to potentially enhance the speed of participant accrual. Later in the workshop, individual workshop speakers and participants discussed in more depth approaches to improve workforce diversity (see Chapter 2), and build trust and sustain long-term relationships with communities and community providers (see Chapter 5).

Improving Community Engagement and Fostering Trust

The need for sustained investments in building communities and maintaining trust was a theme across the breakout discussions. Breakout discussants observed that the clinical trials enterprise seems "piecework" in that generally each trial is set up independently, making it difficult to have a sustainable impact in a given community. The importance of leveraging established partnerships to engage target communities was highlighted in the breakout discussions. The role of community-based participatory research was highlighted, including the need to consider community researchers as part of the clinical research team. Lessons may be learned from the response to the COVID-19 pandemic, which involved leveraging existing skills, resources, and infrastructure within communities (e.g., community-based pharmacies).

ENVISIONING AN OPTIMIZED CLINICAL TRIALS ENTERPRISE THROUGH THE USE OF TECHNOLOGIES

A Perspective on the Use of Digital Technologies: Taking Action for Impact

Califf described the development of COVID-19 vaccines as "a real triumph," but added that the clinical trials enterprise in general did not deliver. "[T]he clinical trials industry … is at the point now where digital transformation is going to have an impact," Califf said. "And the way people handle it will determine the winners and the losers as things shake out." He provided examples of digital disruption in other industries, such as the transformation of photography from film and paper to digital and the movement from video rental to digital streaming, in which the digital disruption was driven by external organizations while the original businesses resisted change (see Steinhubl et al., 2019). He suggested that the clinical trials enterprise embrace the coming digital disruption and adapt technologies to improve clinical research and care.

Califf referred participants to the vision statement by the Clinical Trials Transformation Initiative (CTTI) on transforming clinical trials for 2030, which he said was in line with the focus of this National Academies workshop.[2] He focused his remarks on seven technology-related actions that he said have the potential to transform the field.

Califf suggested that one approach could be to replace human labor through automation, while not replacing human jobs. He observed that

---

[2] See https://ctti-clinicaltrials.org/who_we_are/transforming-trials-2030 (accessed April 13, 2022).

some manual processes in the conduct of clinical trials could be automated, but concerns about regulatory oversight have stalled progress. "We have to move into a regulatory regime that supports and does not inhibit automation," he said. Automation could enhance the efficiency of virtual visits, virtual monitoring, auditing, and statistical process control, for example. Califf asserted that automation could reduce the time spent doing mundane, repetitive tasks and allow trial staff to spend more time on higher value activities, including interacting with clinical trial participants.

Another approach that Califf proposed was to provide digital support that makes the work easier and more fun. Califf offered suggestions for how digital support might enhance the conduct of clinical trials. For example, trial participation can be made more engaging for patients through the use of gamification—the application of game design elements to non-game situations. Decision support tools for clinical trials and clinical practice could help providers delegate some routine health care activities to other staff, which would share the workload across the health care team and enable providers to focus on other priority tasks. The use of passive measurement technologies (with informed consent) can enhance virtual visits and reduce the burden of data collection. Digital support can also enable more home health visits, and "digital phenotypes" can help ensure that the technology used is appropriate for the individual (e.g., some patients might need more personal interaction or might be less technology literate).

A third approach Califf suggested was to scale research in a way that is representative, reliable, and powerful. He said the dependence on manual processes limits the ability to reach populations of potential trial participants. For common chronic diseases, many of those who are eligible for a trial can face barriers to participation, such as not living near a trial site. Rare disease trials can be challenging to enroll in small areas and can require coordination across health systems and geographies. Digital health technologies can enable the conduct of research at the scale needed for studies to be representative, reliable, and adequately powered to produce meaningful data, he said.

A fourth approach Califf suggested was to involve patients and participants directly in research. Digital health technologies can enable direct interaction with patients and potential trial participants to gain input on their priorities, preferences, and concerns (e.g., features of trial design and outcomes of importance to patients). Technology can also enable self-reporting by participants, which Califf said can add depth and context to clinical and functional outcomes measures.

Califf proposed creating communities of learning and research as another approach. Concerns about patient and participant privacy and data integrity have resulted in a system that does not facilitate interaction among the broad range of stakeholders in clinical research, Califf observed. He said it is time to develop communities of learning in the clinical research enterprise.

Califf emphasized the need to integrate research and practice. He noted that the quality of electronic health records (EHR) data and claims data is improving, and standards, common data models, and automated curation methods that are being developed and deployed can help support the advancement of a learning health system.

Lastly, Califf pointed to the use of cloud computing to federate data, information, and knowledge. Technology can be used to optimize the collection, storage, curation, and global sharing of data for regulatory and technology assessment purposes, Califf said. Technology has enabled the ability to "bring the questions to the data," rather than just bring data to the questions, he continued. "[W]e are going to be much better off if we create global datasets that are available, with the proper protections, to a variety of people to try to understand what the data mean and to participate in the research in a direct way," Califf said.

Fundamental Non-Technical Issues to Be Addressed

Several non-technical issues need to be addressed if technologies are to be used to their fullest extent in clinical trials, Califf said. These include the interrelated issues of how to govern the privacy and confidentiality of health-related data; prioritization of clinical studies (and who determines priorities); and how to balance the risks versus the benefits of clinical trial participation.

Ultimately, he said, "Digital technology can either be a rising tide that raises all boats if we make it equitable ... or it can be used much like it is now in most of our health systems ... to segment populations to optimize the situation for some people, particularly those who are already digitally enabled."

Using Technology to Optimize the Clinical Trials Enterprise: Breakout Discussion Highlights

A summary of the points made by individual breakout group participants was provided in plenary session by Celia Witten of the Center for Biologics Evaluation and Research (CBER) at FDA, Sam Roosz of Crescendo Health, Ed Seguine of Clinical Ink, and Jeanne Regnante of the LUNGevity Foundation on behalf of breakout groups. The following topics were highlighted as being of interest for further discussion in subsequent workshop meetings (see Chapter 4). This section is the rapporteurs' summary of the breakout groups reports by Witten, Roosz, Seguine, and Regnante, and should not be construed as reflecting any group. All suggestions and proposals are reported for discussion purposes only.

The Use of Digital Health Technologies in Trials

Breakout participants discussed the need to intentionally consider whether the use of digital health technologies in clinical trials would be deployed as a tool to more effectively mine data from communities (i.e., with limited return of information or benefit to the community) versus being used as a tool to work more collaboratively with patients and communities (e.g., to reduce the burden of trial participation and return information back to individuals and communities, and to build value and transparency in the research enterprise). The acceptability of technologies and innovative methodologies in regulatory submissions may not be clearly established, so breakout participants suggested that guidance for industry from regulators might be needed so that sponsors can more confidently deploy these technologies in trials. Participants also discussed the need for training of clinical operations staff to ensure they are confident in the use of current and new technologies for clinical trials. The lack of clear and consistent terminology across industry regarding the use of technologies in trials was also raised. Breakout participants highlighted the need to disseminate information about initiatives and best practices for the use of technologies in clinical trials. The importance of applying lessons from the response to the COVID-19 pandemic to the use of technology in clinical research was also a recurring theme of discussion (see Chapter 4).

Technology and Trial Participants

The role of technology in trial recruitment was discussed, including the use of advanced analytics to identify potential participants from underrepresented groups, and engaging and establishing relationships with communities through the use of social media. The need to better leverage the power of communication was highlighted, including communication campaigns to educate the public about the benefits of trials and trial technologies. It was observed that access to technology tools varies across communities. Breakout participants discussed the value of investing in access to technology resources within communities, with a focus on technology that would fit into trial participants' daily lives.

Data Collection and Sharing

Breakout participants discussed the need for harmonization of data collection and tools that can facilitate data sharing and translation across data systems, so that data collection efforts do not hinder existing workflows and practices. The need to engage patients in identifying the outcomes of interest to them first, before designing the study, was also raised. Participants discussed the importance of responsibly and transparently sharing data from clinical trials with communities to build public trust in clinical research and add value back to the community.

ENVISIONING A MORE RESILIENT, SUSTAINABLE, AND TRANSPARENT CLINICAL TRIALS ENTERPRISE

A Perspective on the State of Clinical Trials in 2021

The clinical research enterprise primarily serves the needs of three key stakeholder groups: sponsors, patients, and societies, Levy said.[3] Clinical research is conducted by the industry sponsors, who seek to improve the speed, efficiency, and success rates of their trials. At the same time, it is important to remember that clinical research is ultimately conducted for the benefit of the patients and for communities impacted by the costs and burdens of disease. Each stakeholder group has its own distinct interests which, he observed, can be in conflict to some extent (i.e., the interest of one might be only satisfied at the expense of another). However, Levy said, "what the pandemic taught us … is that a greater focus on the needs of patients and societies is, in fact, consistent with the industry's needs for greater efficiency and productivity and therefore we can transform the clinical research enterprise in a way that benefits all parties, including industry." Levy considered the current and future states of research from the perspective of each stakeholder group.

Sponsor Perspective: Enhance Efficiencies

Clinical research is a high-risk, costly, complex enterprise with poor success rates and low return on investment, Levy said. He explained that, in the absence of price increases, such an industry can only survive in a capital-rich environment. From a sponsor perspective, increasing operational efficiencies is essential. Levy outlined four areas for opportunity:

- Continuous process improvement could yield improvements in efficiency which, while incremental, could compound over time. Improved process efficiency also benefits patients by, for example,

---

[3] Levy noted that the opinions expressed in his presentation are solely his own and do not necessarily represent those of his employer or any other party.

reducing site workload, thereby allowing sites to focus more on patients than process.
- Platform trials, adaptive trial designs, and the use of historical clinical trial comparator data could increase trial efficiencies. Patients can benefit as well, Levy said. For example, use of a historical comparator means that participants are less likely to receive an ineffective clinical comparator.
- Trial simplification could result in cost savings (e.g., large outcomes trials following on the initial registration trial).
- Substitution of real-world evidence for evidence gathered in the course of traditional clinical trials could increase trial efficiency. Levy said he expects increased attention and use of real-world evidence in the coming years.

Levy pointed out that improving industry efficiency may also help reduce the burden of trial participation for patients and increase the volume of reliable and relevant data available to support evidence-based decision making on the part of stakeholders across the clinical trials enterprise.

Looking beyond operational efficiencies, Levy suggested that the expanding use of data and technology in trial design and execution will significantly improve the speed, efficiency, and success of clinical trials in the coming decade. Real-world data collected in health care settings can help provide a more complete picture of local patient characteristics and standards of care, which can be used to refine eligibility criteria and site selection, making trial enrollment more efficient and predictable. The increasing availability of patient-level genomic and proteomic data will enable identification of patients who would be most likely to benefit from the investigational intervention. This would enable smaller, faster studies, Levy said, and increase value for patients and society. Improved analytics, artificial intelligence, and machine learning can be applied to generate faster, more rigorous systematic reviews to inform the development of research questions and study designs, and to screening incoming clinical trial data for safety and other signals. There is also potential for new data collection approaches, such as passive data collection by wearable devices, to expand in scope over the coming decade and contribute to improved trial design and execution.

Patient Perspective

Levy outlined some patient-centered elements that he believes will be parts of future clinical trials:

DEFINING THE VISION

- "Patients will routinely participate in the design of clinical trials," Levy said.
- Trials will be more accessible through increased selection of sites in community settings, and through the increased use of remote trial conduct methods that were more broadly deployed and validated during the COVID-19 pandemic (see Figure 2-1).
- Adaptive trial designs can reduce the amount of non-informative testing to which participants are subjected, and platform trials can increase the likelihood of participants receiving an effective therapy.
- Advances in genomics and proteomics will allow for tailoring of treatments to individual patient needs and increase the probability of patient benefit.

"All these changes, which are made in the interest of patients, will benefit sponsors by improving recruitment, retention, and data quality,"

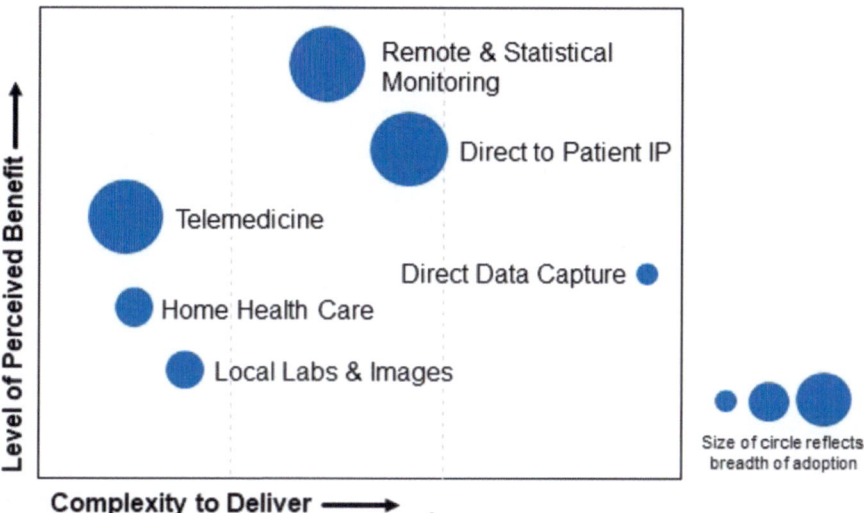

FIGURE 2-1 One sponsor's qualitative impression of the adoption and impact of remote approaches on the conduct of clinical trials during a pandemic.
NOTES: Approaches adopted (to varying degrees as indicated by circle size) included telemedicine, remote and statistical monitoring, shipment of investigational product (IP) directly to patients, home health care, local collection of laboratory and imaging data, and direct data capture. Levy noted that the effort expended to deploy these approaches was generally acceptable to the sponsor and enabled the sponsor to safely continue and complete the study during the COVID-19 pandemic.
SOURCE: Levy presentation, January 26, 2021.

Levy added. As an example, he described Amgen's approach to end-to-end patient engagement in the drug development process. Prior to the start of Phase 1, Amgen gathers patient input on their unmet treatment needs. When a target had been identified, patients provide input on their desired attributes for the products, and specify elements of the study design that would enable or encourage them to participate (e.g., dosing regimens, outcomes measures). The patient voice is also increasingly included in sponsor interactions with regulatory authorities and payers.

Societal Perspective

Levy observed that not enough clinical trial data are available on minority populations because of the underrepresentation of minority participants in clinical trials. He noted that participating in clinical trials "is a problem with deep historical roots" for many African Americans, and added that limited access to clinical trials in general compounds the barriers to participation for many underrepresented populations. The competitive model, by default, can limit the sharing of clinical trial data, and drives biopharmaceutical investment toward areas where incentives are greatest. This can lead to investments that are not aligned with societal need, leading to a lack of trust in the clinical research enterprise, Levy said.

There is opportunity for improvement in the value that the clinical trials enterprise delivers to societies, Levy said. He listed a few steps toward a future state that better promotes health equity and public trust:

- The balance between collaboration and competition should be reset to maintain incentives for innovation while expanding the scope of precompetitive collaboration and data sharing.
- A modified incentive system could help drive investments toward clinical research that is in better alignment with public health priorities, which in turn can help build public trust in the enterprise.
- A systematic effort is needed to increase diversity among trial participants. Levy suggested, "Clinical trial diversity can be increased. We already know how. What is most needed is simply the will and the discipline to systematically apply existing methods."

The COVID-19 pandemic has been a driver of change in clinical research and health care and has led to increased sharing of data and other proprietary information (AstraZeneca, 2020; COVID R&D Alliance, 2021; FDA, 2020a; Janssen Vaccines and Prevention, 2020; Moderna TX, 2020; Pfizer, 2020; TransCelerate, 2020). For example, the major COVID-19 vaccine trial protocols were publicly posted, which Levy said would previously have been "unthinkable." The public disclosure of COVID-19 vaccine trial data drew attention to the issue of diversity in trial populations and has fostered discussions of minority underrepresentation in these trials. One notable example of this type of collaboration, Levy said, is the COVID R&D Alliance of major biopharmaceutical companies, which is focused on accelerating development of therapies for COVID-19 though repurposing, trial acceleration, data sharing, and pandemic preparedness. Another example is TransCelerate BioPharma, Inc., a nonprofit collaborative established in 2012 by the major biopharmaceutical companies to advance clinical research. In response to COVID-19, TransCelerate developed and launched a platform for sharing patient-level data from COVID-19 trials among researchers to inform future trial design and conduct (e.g., refining eligibility criteria, optimizing endpoints for assay sensitivity).

The interests of the sponsors, patients, and societies are not necessarily in conflict, Levy concluded. A more patient- and society-focused clinical research enterprise can also be more efficient and productive for industry trial sponsors.

Building a More Resilient, Sustainable, and Transparent Clinical Trials Enterprise: Breakout Discussion Highlights

A summary of the points made by individual breakout group participants was provided in plenary session by Clay Johnston of the Dell Medical School, Peyton Howell of Parexel, Jeanne Regnante of the LUNGevity Foundation, and Celia Witten of CBER at FDA on behalf of each of the four breakout groups. The following topics were highlighted as being of interest for further discussion in subsequent workshop meetings (see Chapter 5). This section is the rapporteurs' summary of the breakout group reports by Johnston, Howell, Regnante, and Witten, and should not be construed as reflecting any group. All suggestions and proposals are reported for discussion purposes only.

Moving Toward Community-Based Trials

Participants discussed ways to better integrate clinical research and routine health care. In the wake of the COVID-19 pandemic and the need for the clinical trials enterprise to be better prepared for the next pandemic, there may be motivation for investments to improve the clinical trials enterprise. Participants discussed the creation of a clinical trials network that is community based, which could quickly transition from routine trials for chronic conditions to trials needed to respond to the next public health emergency. It was observed, however, that many communities lack the infrastructure needed for efficient participation in current clinical trials.

Approaches to address systemic racism and how to bring clinical trials to communities were discussed. Breakout discussants shared ideas for engaging trusted community members as brokers, involving the community in the development of trial networks, and fostering a clinical trials workforce that reflects the patients in the communities they serve.

Workforce and Workflow

Participants discussed the need to develop career paths and incentives for primary care and community-based physicians to act as clinical trial investigators in multicenter trials. Similarly, incentives for academic investigators to participate in large platform trials versus initiating their own smaller trials were discussed. Breakout discussants emphasized the need to fund the conduct and expansion of community-based participatory research and training and to provide incentives for community-based researchers. Workflow issues were also discussed, such as the pressures on clinical investigators to meet the competing demands of clinical trials and health care delivery.

Evidence Generation and Regulatory Review

The generation of quality data to support regulatory review was a key topic of interest. Participants discussed the role of institutional review boards (IRBs) in preventing uninformative trials from moving forward, and how enhanced coordination between regulators and industry sponsors might help ensure that data generated through novel methods will be acceptable for regulatory review and approval. The use of real-world data in clinical trials was highlighted as a means to bridge clinical research and health care delivery, and the need for standardized definitions of data elements in EHRs was noted. Breakout discussants suggested there may be lessons learned based on the UK RECOVERY Trial (see Chapter 5) and other ongoing efforts that have successfully coordinated clinical trials and enabled the sharing of standardized trial data.

3

Enhancing Outcomes in a More Person-Centered and Inclusive Clinical Trials Enterprise

> **Highlights of Key Points Made by Individual Speakers**
>
> - Science benefits from diverse participation in studies that can lead to new discoveries and treatment approaches. However, the clinical trials enterprise has not evolved to reflect the population it now serves. (Pérez-Stable)
> - Collecting input from patients on trial design, including the consent process, can lead to more patient-centered trials and better participant recruitment and retention. (Araojo, O'Boyle, Pérez-Stable)
> - The response to the COVID-19 pandemic shows that inclusivity in trials can be achieved when there is appropriate attention to overcoming barriers through early-stage planning, appropriate site selection, and community engagement. (Araojo)
> - Relationships with community organizations should be equitable partnerships and nurtured over the long term. (Buchanan)
> - The vision for health care in 2030 is built around "achieving optimal outcomes with as little added burden to the patient as possible." (Metcalf)
> - Stakeholders across the clinical trials enterprise need to better explain the usefulness and value of clinical research for the practice of medicine and clinical care. (Anderson)

This segment of the four-part workshop focused on transforming the clinical trials enterprise to be more person-centered, inclusive, and equitable by 2030. Participants discussed priorities and actions for achieving this goal and how to engage stakeholders, including the public, in this effort.

THE ROAD TO 2030: PERSPECTIVES FROM THE FIELD

Frontline Experience: A Panel Discussion

In this session, panelists shared their perspectives on what is needed for the clinical trials enterprise to move toward greater person-centeredness over the coming decade. Panelists included Eliseo Pérez-Stable, director of the National Institute on Minority Health and Health Disparities (NIMHD) at the National Institutes of Health (NIH); Richardae Araojo, associate commissioner for Minority Health and director of the Office of Minority Health and Health Equity (OMHHE) at FDA; and Megan O'Boyle, principal investigator of the Phelan-McDermid Syndrome Registry. The session was moderated by Esther Krofah.

The Rationale for Inclusiveness

Pérez-Stable said increasing the inclusiveness of clinical trials is a priority. "Having a diverse sample in a clinical research trial is good science," Pérez-Stable said. "There are questions that will be left unanswered if we stay with the easiest-to-recruit participants in a clinical research trial." Furthermore, some groups experience disproportionate burdens from particular diseases. For example, he said that because COVID-19 is disproportionately impacting African American and Latino individuals, it may make sense to oversample them for related clinical trials. He acknowledged the challenge of achieving balanced representation in every study, but said that having at least some diverse participation in studies can lead to new discoveries and treatment approaches.

Araojo mentioned the 2012 FDA Safety and Innovation Act (FDASIA), which directed the agency to study the participation and analysis of demographic subgroups in clinical trials and to create a plan to support inclusive clinical trials.[1] One product of FDASIA was the FDA Center for Drug Evaluation and Research's Drug Trials Snapshots program. Araojo shared some specific findings from a recent Snapshots report summarizing participant demographics in clinical trials of new products from

---

[1] See https://www.fda.gov/regulatory-information/food-and-drug-administration-safety-and-innovation-act-fdasia/fdasia-section-907-inclusion-demographic-subgroups-clinical-trials (accessed July 1, 2021).

2015 through 2019.[2] Of the nearly 300,000 trial participants during this time frame (from both U.S. and ex-U.S. trial sites), 76 percent were white, 11 percent were Asian, 7 percent were Black or African American, and about 1 percent were American Indian or Alaska Native (5 percent were designated as other). When only participants enrolled at U.S. sites were assessed (about 102,000), the demographics shifted to 16 percent Black or African American, 2 percent Asian, and 1 percent American Indian or Alaska Native (FDA, 2020b).

O'Boyle observed that there is little diversity in clinical trials for rare diseases, unless the disease is known to be highly prevalent in a particular ethnic or racial group. She suggested that diversity in rare disease trials could be improved if providers referred more patients for genetic testing.

The Role of the U.S. Food and Drug Administration

OMHHE at FDA "works to protect and promote the health of racial and ethnic minority, underrepresented, and underserved populations [through] research, outreach, and communication that works toward addressing health disparities," Araojo said.[3] Activities within the agency's current authorities include, for example, supporting intramural and extramural research; implementing culturally and linguistically appropriate strategies, tools, programs, initiatives, and campaigns; and issuing guidance documents. Improving diversity in clinical trials is a key priority for FDA, and Araojo referred participants to a recently released guidance for industry, *Enhancing the Diversity of Clinical Trial Populations—Eligibility Criteria, Enrollment Practices, and Trial Designs*.[4] The guidance addresses methods to improve trial recruitment so those enrolled reflect those who will ultimately use the product being studied.

Araojo said FDA is committed to "consistent, continued, bidirectional community engagement" to advance inclusiveness and to help overcome the barriers to more representative participation of racial and ethnic minority populations in clinical trials. The agency will continue its efforts to reduce the burden of trial participation, and will apply the lessons learned, as appropriate, during the COVID-19 response about the use of new technologies, tools, techniques, real-world data, and other advances.

---

[2] For the *2015–2019 Drug Trials Snapshots Summary Report*, see https://www.fda.gov/media/143592/download (accessed July 1, 2021).

[3] For more information about OMHHE at FDA, see https://www.fda.gov/about-fda/office-commissioner/office-minority-health-and-health-equity (accessed July 1, 2021).

[4] See https://www.fda.gov/regulatory-information/search-fda-guidance-documents/enhancing-diversity-clinical-trial-populations-eligibility-criteria-enrollment-practices-and-trial (accessed July 1, 2021).

Engaging the Community to Reduce Barriers to Enrollment

O'Boyle spoke from her perspective as the principal investigator of the Phelan-McDermid Syndrome Registry and as the parent of a child with a rare genetic syndrome. She described the current clinical trials enterprise as out of alignment with the way people use and share personal data in 2021. IRBs are providing protections that participants do not necessarily want, and required consents often do not allow participants to share identified data, she said. Furthermore, much of what is included in consent forms is unnecessary, frightening to participants, or redundant. Forms are lengthy and seem to be written for the benefit of corporate lawyers rather than patients, O'Boyle said. "Short, concise, honest" forms are needed, and patient groups should be approached to review consent forms before IRB approval. O'Boyle said that sponsors should also seek input from patient groups on protocols and schedules (e.g., Would treatment be better tolerated before or after a meal? Will travel to appointments be a financial burden?). Patient input can inform the development of more patient-centered trials, which can lead to better participant retention.

O'Boyle said that time, money, and lives are being wasted as a result of "overprotection" by IRBs and a lack of inclusion of diverse patients in studies. She stressed that this message must come from patients and research advocacy organizations. Any effort by the researchers to address this would appear self-serving. Patient communities need education about clinical trials so they are empowered to speak up and communicate to trial sponsors their interests and concerns about protocols and consent forms.

Pérez-Stable emphasized the importance of understanding patient needs when designing trial procedures and the consent form. He agreed that consent forms need to be more user-friendly for participants, not just in length and content, but also language and reading level. Protocols or consent forms that are not acceptable or understandable to patients can be a barrier to recruiting a diverse population, and experience has shown that community engagement is an effective method for developing long-term connections with diverse populations.

Araojo highlighted the need for engaging patient advocacy groups to learn how to make trials less burdensome with regard to trial design, logistics, recruitment, and retention; engaging cultural ambassadors, faith-based organizations, and trusted leaders in the community; and eliminating language barriers. Community engagement is not just informing the community, it is also understanding their needs with regard to trial participation.

Another barrier to recruitment is a general lack of awareness of the availability of clinical trials, Araojo said. With COVID-19, the public was aware that trials were being launched and that volunteers were needed, and that diverse participation was especially needed due to the disproportionate impact of COVID-19 in racial and ethnic minority communities. A lesson from the response to the COVID-19 pandemic is that inclusivity in trials can be achieved when there is appropriate attention to overcoming barriers through early-stage planning, appropriate site selection, and community engagement.

Krofah asked panelists to comment on the concerns that including patients in discussions of trial design and working to increase diverse participation slows the process and adds expense. O'Boyle said that *failure* to recruit or retain trial participants slows the process and increases expense. "If you do not design [trials] with the patients and families in mind, then you are not going to retain them," she said. She advocated for engaging with patients and their caregivers even earlier, prior to selecting a target and defining product attributes or delivery mechanisms, to understand what their most pressing disease-related concerns and quality-of-life issue are.

Best Practices

Pérez-Stable said that planning for representative trial participation should be done early, and he suggested that experts might reach out to the contract research organizations recruiting in areas with minority populations to motivate them. He shared his experience working with the Operation Warp Speed[5] leadership to increase their outreach to diverse communities. One of the COVID-19 vaccine sponsors, for example, created a website for people to register their interest in joining the trial. However, participants from all demographics did not visit the website in proportionate numbers right away, he said, and recruiters initially failed to reach out to many people from diverse communities who did register. The sponsor did understand the importance of diverse enrollment, he continued, and ultimately paused recruitment of white participants to achieve better representation of minority populations.

Pérez-Stable emphasized the importance of finding the right messenger to reach out to diverse communities. Too often recruiters believe that minorities are not interested in clinical trials, he said, or that they will only participate in trials if a religious leader or a celebrity or athlete endorses the trial. The most powerful messengers are actually local doctors, nurses, and community leaders who can speak in plain language to community members. The panelists also emphasized the importance of investing in

---

[5] Operation Warp Speed was a public–private partnership to accelerate the development of vaccines for COVID-19.

culturally tailored and linguistically competent messages and literature to share with patients from many backgrounds.

Krofah noted that community outreach and efforts to educate the public about clinical trials are chronically underfunded. Pérez-Stable observed that academic clinical research has been gradually moving toward early community engagement and said that industry has come to understand the value of investing in community engagement. He cited the COVID-19 Prevention Network (CoVPN)[6] run by the National Institute of Allergy and Infectious Diseases as one positive example of COVID-19 clinical trials recruiting diverse participants. Pérez-Stable added that the NIH Community Engagement Alliance (CEAL) Against COVID-19 Disparities[7] is investing community engagement, providing resources, and partnering with communities to develop and disseminate accurate information about COVID-19 disease, clinical trials, and vaccination.

THE ROAD TO 2030: VISIONS OF WHAT IS POSSIBLE

In this session, Silas Buchanan, chief executive officer of the Institute for eHealth Equity, shared several examples of how the Institute for eHealth Equity is working to create equitable partnerships with community organizations. Marilyn Metcalf, senior director of patient engagement at GlaxoSmithKline, discussed the potential for technology tools to improve patient outcomes and reduce patient burdens. Margaret Anderson, consulting managing director of strategy and analytics at Deloitte, described lessons from health movements of the past that can be brought forward to effect change for the future. The session was moderated by Luther Clark, deputy chief patient officer and global director for scientific, medical, and patient perspective at Merck & Co.

Forging Equitable Partnerships with Community-Based Organizations[8]

"A more inclusive clinical trials enterprise in 2030 will largely be defined by the number of equitable partnerships … created with underserved, faith, and community-based organizations," Buchanan began.

---

[6] For more information about CoVPN, see https://coronaviruspreventionnetwork.org (accessed August 3, 2021).

[7] For more information about the NIH CEAL program, see https://covid19community.nih.gov (accessed July 20, 2021).

[8] This presentation is based on a blog post titled *Driving Towards a More Inclusive Clinical Trials Enterprise by 2030: Action Without Strategy Is Aimless and Strategy Without Action Is Powerless*, available at https://www.healthaffairs.org/do/10.1377/hblog20210503.43985/full (accessed July 1, 2021).

This strategy for inclusiveness depends on building trusted relationships with the leaders of these organizations, whom he said serve as conduits between underserved community members and the health care system. These types of community-based organizations have a wealth of experience addressing social determinants of health, Buchanan noted. Religious organizations, for example, have a long history of addressing food insecurity and other personal needs (e.g., soup kitchens, food pantries, clothing drives, transportation to health care appointments, daycare and after-school programs, adult education/GED classes). As discussed by workshop speaker Terris King, formerly of CMS (see Chapter 2), conversations about health also take place at barbershops and beauty salons, which are trusted community institutions where people feel safe discussing their personal concerns. Buchanan observed that the clinical trials enterprise has long underestimated the importance of equitably partnering with these trusted organizations as emissaries to the community. He cautioned, however, that it is not as simple as just reaching out to a church for a particular clinical trial. These relationships need to be nurtured over time.

As an example of how to begin reaching out to underserved communities, Buchanan described launching a Healthy Eating Active Living (HEAL) campaign. With a grant from the Aetna Foundation, the Institute for eHealth Equity partnered with five churches in Atlanta, Georgia; Dallas, Texas; and Columbus, Ohio, to co-create a HEAL campaign. Buchanan emphasized that they did not arrive with a fully developed campaign and tell the community what to do. Rather, decisions about aspects such as content, language, and images were community-driven, and endorsed by the participating faith-based organizations.

The campaign was facilitated by SMS text messaging. After the pastor spoke briefly to the congregation about health, they could text "healthy" to a short code phone number and begin answering a series of demographic and health-related questions. The HEAL campaign then messaged the 2,500 participating community members three times each week with additional information and questions. Over the course of 6 months, the response rate to the questions was 43 percent and, importantly, Buchanan said, no one left the program. Key elements of success, he said, were having each pastor's blessing to launch the campaign, and gathering feedback and discussing next steps in weekly private meetings with the health ministry teams. Buchanan noted that about 35 percent of African Methodist Episcopal (AME) churches have a health ministry team, which usually includes members of the congregation who are current and retired nurses and doctors. Decisions about the HEAL campaign were driven by them as the experts on their community.

The relationships built through the HEAL campaign led to a partnership with the AME Church to launch AMECHealth.org,[9] which Buchanan said is now the official channel for dissemination of health information for the AME Church. The website includes both publicly available information and a password-protected social network for the leadership of AME congregations, which the Institute for eHealth Equity uses to facilitate equitable collaboration and data sharing for health campaigns. He noted that many major health programs designed to reach African Americans through faith-based organizations collect data, but do not share data back in a lay format that the organizations can use (e.g., to apply for grants).

The Institute for eHealth Equity is also launching Our Healthy Community teams, a social network for community-based organizations designed to "shorten the distance" between the community and the clinical trials enterprise, health care providers, payers, and other stakeholders in health. Buchanan added that the Institute for eHealth Equity was recently selected by the Morehouse School of Medicine to participate on the National Advisory Board for the National COVID-19 Resiliency Network. They are developing a co-branded campaign with Morehouse, again working directly with faith-based organizations to ensure their input is included.

"What we are most interested in," Buchanan concluded, "is helping to equitably connect all stakeholders, helping recruit more principal investigators of color, and building something that acknowledges the past while moving together toward the future."

Achieving Improved Outcomes While Reducing Patient Burden

Metcalf shared a vision for health care in 2030 developed in collaboration with Rob Weker, a patient advocate, and based on input from patients.[10] In this vision, a patient's well-being would be monitored, to the extent they desired, making use of artificial intelligence and digital networking to provide comprehensive, proactive health services to the patient and the caregiver. Health care would ideally encompass early detection of disease, shared decision making about options, psychosocial support, expert medical care, and financial support, Metcalf said, with the goal of "achieving optimal outcomes with as little added burden to the patient as possible."

The technical capabilities to achieve this vision exist or are being developed, Metcalf said. She pointed out, however, that patients who

---

[9] For more information, see http://amechealth.org (accessed July 20, 2021).
[10] This presentation is based on a blog post titled *Transforming Clinical Trials: A New Vision for 2030*, available at https://www.healthaffairs.org/do/10.1377/hblog20210503.897529/full (accessed July 1, 2021).

have access to specialty medical facilities and have comprehensive insurance coverage are most likely to benefit. It is important to "consider the patients who are not well insured, who do not have physicians, or whose physicians do not have familiarity with or access to clinical trials and cutting-edge therapies," Metcalf said.

Issues such as infrastructure, access, equity, and privacy are systemic issues that cannot be addressed effectively by one segment of the health system in isolation, she added. Furthermore, technical capability alone will not achieve this vision for 2030. Technologies are tools, and their accessibility and appeal to patients varies.

Achieving this vision requires an integrated health care system with shared purpose and shared information. The translation of research into clinical practice can be supported by prioritizing patient involvement in drug R&D and regulatory decision making when it comes to early disease detection, disease management, and treatment, Metcalf said.

Metcalf referred participants to a prior workshop of the National Academies' Forum on Drug Discovery, Development, and Translation on Advancing the Science of Patient Input in Medical Product Research and Development[11] (NASEM, 2018). Discussions at that workshop highlighted the importance of designing trials from the start with patient needs and preferences in mind, and gathering input on participant trial experiences, including the experiences of participants who drop out of studies. Although some progress has been made in forging closer partnerships between patients and the health system, much work still needs to be done. "Creating an equitable person-centered health care system is not only possible, but absolutely necessary for the well-being of all people," Metcalf concluded.

Advocating for Change: Learning from Past Movements That Changed Policy and Practice

Anderson reflected on how the current clinical trials system was formed by events of the past. In particular, she described how unethical practices in medical research, such as the U.S. Public Health Service Syphilis Study at Tuskegee, and the widespread use of Henrietta Lacks's cells without her knowledge or consent, led to mistrust of the medical research system. Citing work by the Pew Research Center, Anderson shared data showing how public trust in the scientific community has remained fairly stable since the 1970s, while public trust in government

---

[11] For more information on this workshop, see https://www.nationalacademies.org/our-work/advancing-the-science-of-patient-input-in-medical-product-rd-towards-a-research-agenda--a-workshop (accessed July 20, 2021).

has declined steeply in the same time period.[12,13] Moving forward, she said that stakeholders across the clinical trials enterprise need to better explain the usefulness and value of clinical research for the practice of medicine and clinical care. In doing so, it is important to remember that "there is deep pain throughout the research system. These are real people, real lives, real diseases. It is important for us to honor that," Anderson said.

Understanding the past is necessary to develop the solutions needed for the future, and Anderson described several examples of movements that changed policy and practice in health care. In the late 1980s, during the early days of the HIV/AIDS epidemic, activists took an "outside/inside" approach to effecting change by staging large public demonstrations outside that demanded attention from government, while also working with science and policy experts to propose specific policy changes from inside organizations. This strategy was also deployed by the Society for Women's Health Research in the mid-1990s to mandate the inclusion of women in clinical trials. For the inside component, they approached female members of Congress to call for a U.S. Government Accountability Office review of the status of inclusion of women and minorities in research, the results of which helped to facilitate policy changes.

Anderson suggested that a similar strategy could be used for achieving and maintaining accountability for more person-centered clinical trials. Building off the movements described above, a range of organizations and actions have been driving change toward patient-centric clinical trials over time, for example, venture philanthropy organizations and foundations that fund research (e.g., the Cystic Fibrosis Foundation), patient cohorts (e.g., PatientsLikeMe, All of Us), nonprofit research organizations (e.g., Patient-Centered Outcomes Research Institute [PCORI]), agencies (e.g., FDA), and legislation (e.g., the 21st Century Cures Act). Anderson pointed out that these activities moved forward while information and methodologies about patient-centricity were still emerging. There was the will to seek change, she said.

In closing, Anderson listed some of the lessons to take forward.

- Meeting people where they are.
- Taking action without fear ("passion plus fearlessness equals change").
- Using an outside/inside strategy to exert pressure on the system.

---

[12] See https://www.pewresearch.org/politics/2021/05/17/public-trust-in-government-1958-2021 (accessed April 13, 2022).

[13] See https://www.pewresearch.org/fact-tank/2020/08/27/public-confidence-in-scientists-has-remained-stable-for-decades (accessed April 13, 2022).

- Gathering a coalition of the willing. "[Think] broadly about who else needs to be brought [into the clinical trials enterprise] and give them assignments," she said.
- Using disruption as a wedge (e.g., leverage the lessons from technology use in the COVID-19 pandemic response).
- Providing appropriate resources and funding for those organizations that are doing the work and reaching out to communities.
- Developing a pipeline of diverse scientists, clinical researchers, and health care providers.

Short-Term Goals to Foster a More Person-Centered and Inclusive Clinical Trials Enterprise: Panel and Breakout Discussion Highlights

Following the panel discussion, workshop participants were divided into virtual Zoom breakout rooms to consider short-term, tangible, and measurable goals and actions that could help ensure a more person-centered and inclusive clinical trials enterprise, and to discuss technologies, tools, and techniques that could be used to enhance inclusiveness and equity in clinical trials. Upon reconvening in plenary session, Krofah and several participants reflected on the panel and breakout group discussions and highlighted the following themes:

- **Investing in community outreach and engagement.** Relationships with the community need to be cultivated and maintained. Participants discussed funding community-based organizations, providing education and training for community members and leaders, compensating community leaders and partners for their time, and returning value to the community, Krofah reported.
- **Educating the community about clinical trial opportunities.** Jacqueline Alikhanni, patient ambassador at PCORI and trial participant, suggested that many patients would participate in clinical trials if they were better informed about what clinical trials are, what opportunities are available, and how to enroll. Educating communities about trials, especially communities of color, would help to foster trust, she said, and could help to overcome reservations about participating in trials that have resulted from a long history of negative experiences with the medical establishment.
- **Engaging patients at the beginning of the trial process to ensure that participation is meaningful.** For example, patients should be asked to provide input on therapeutic targets and outcomes of importance to them, and on the acceptability of elements of protocols and consent forms, Krofah reported. The need to balance what

is meaningful to trial participants versus what is legally required in consent forms was noted.
- **Rethinking data-sharing practices.** Krofah summarized a point made by O'Boyle that, in some cases, trial participants might prefer to have informed consent agreements that permit sharing of identifiable information. Information not related to health is being shared constantly, such as with social media or streaming services. Some trial participants might choose to similarly share their health information if it could help develop meaningful treatments more efficiently.
- **Clearly defining what is meant by community.** "Different stakeholders define community differently," Krofah said. Identifying trusted leaders in the defined community who can be partners and spokespersons is also important.
- **Identifying appropriate metrics to assess progress in establishing a more person-centered and inclusive clinical trials enterprise.** End-to-end visibility is needed with regard to diverse patient enrollment across trials while still preserving patient privacy and conforming to regulations, Krofah said.
- **Mentoring principal investigators.** Elena Rios of the National Hispanic Medical Association said that physicians involved in research need to serve as mentors to the next generation of clinical trial investigators. She added that many experienced investigators are associated with academic health centers while many new investigators are community based.
- **Considering social determinants of health in inclusiveness.** Barbara Bierer, director of the Multi-Regional Clinical Trials Center of Brigham and Women's Hospital and Harvard University, said that information on social determinants of health is needed to inform diverse trial enrollment efforts, and that good, quick indicators of social determinants of health are needed for use in data collection (versus extensive, often uncomfortable, questioning of patients). Krofah agreed and added that "the full experience of an individual [influences] whether or not they even have the opportunity to understand and participate in clinical trials and research."
- **Developing a national, cooperative effort to educate stakeholders about inclusivity in clinical trials.** Bierer suggested that the National Academies consider which aspects of improving inclusivity might be addressed cooperatively, at a national level, rather than organizations developing uncoordinated, individual efforts to educate about inclusivity.

Long-Term Goals to Foster a More Person-Centered and Inclusive Clinical Trials Enterprise: Panel and Breakout Discussion Highlights

Workshop participants considered longer-term, tangible, and measurable goals and actions that could ensure a more person-centered and inclusive clinical trials enterprise, and discussed technologies, tools, and techniques that could be used to enhance inclusiveness and equity in clinical trials. Upon reconvening in plenary session, Clark reflected on the panel and breakout group discussions and highlighted the following themes:

- **Acting with urgency.** Although the breakout discussants were charged with discussing actions and goals for the next 10 years, Clark reported that several breakout discussants emphasized that the importance of the issues warranted quick actions to begin making progress toward the stated goal and meeting any interim milestones as soon as possible.
- **Focusing on earlier, broader, and consistent community engagement.** The importance of community engagement was a key theme of the discussions, Clark said, including the benefits for both researchers and participants of engaging communities earlier in the clinical trial process. It was suggested that local health equity initiatives are an underused resource for continuous community engagement, and that clinical trials should be connected to these groups.
- **Moving the clinical trials enterprise into health care settings.** Breakout participants discussed the importance of developing robust clinical trial networks within communities, and investing in community-based trial infrastructure for the long term. Approaches might include: establishing sustainable funding models for community health workers, providing training opportunities for individuals working across the health care team to help patients make more informed decisions about trial participation, and sustaining long-term relationships between community leaders and the health care teams.
- **Advancing the consent process.** Participants discussed ways in which technology could be used to make consent forms and the consent process more interactive, more meaningful and patient friendly, and potentially virtual.
- **Collecting information on social determinants of health.** In addition to the usual demographic information, better information is needed on the social determinants of health impacting potential

trial participants. Collecting the latter information should not create additional burden for the trial participant, Clark said, and breakout discussants suggested that the clinical trials enterprise connect with community partners that are already collecting this information as they work to address these issues.

- **Identifying the problems that could be solved with technology.** Breakout participants discussed how technology could help overcome many of the barriers to more person-centered and inclusive clinical trials, Clark reported. There was discussion of the need to address the "digital divide" and to ensure that patients with limited access to technology or technology literacy are not excluded. General areas discussed in which digital health technologies could help improve patient-centeredness and inclusiveness included
- **Raising awareness about clinical trials.** Technology can be an effective tool to disseminate reliable, high-quality, credible information about clinical trials, Clark said. It was also noted that technology can be leveraged to help foster trust in the clinical trials enterprise if trusted community voices are delivering the messages.
- **Increasing access to clinical trials.** Breakout participants discussed how to leverage technology to decentralize clinical trials and expand the population that can participate. Mobile technologies can be used to reach those living in rural and remote areas and others who face barriers to traveling to a clinical trial site, Clark said. Cell phones, for example, are now widely available even in the most remote parts of the world.

REFLECTIONS ON ACHIEVING PERSON-CENTERED AND INCLUSIVE TRIALS

Steven Galson and Krofah noted that an underlying theme throughout this part of the workshop was that the issues of person-centeredness and inclusivity in clinical trials have been discussed for decades and the time has come to take action, employ new approaches, and make progress. To close this part of the workshop, they summarized some of the key messages they heard during the discussions.

Person-Centeredness and Inclusiveness

- "If the patients are not at the center of our work, then who is?" Galson said, paraphrasing O'Boyle. To move forward, it is necessary to understand where and why there has been resistance to engaging patients and their caregivers in the clinical trials process.

- Communities need information about what clinical trials are and the advantages of participating, Galson summarized. It is a misperception that certain minority populations do not want to participate in clinical trials.
- Ease of recruitment often drives who is recruited for a given clinical study and, as discussed by Pérez-Stable, this does not represent the best science.
- The population enrolled in a trial does not necessarily reflect the population most burdened by the disease under investigation, Galson said. A summary of participant demographics that was discussed by Araojo showed that 16 percent of trial participants in the United States were Black or African American and 2 percent were Asian.
- There is also a need to engage and prepare a more diverse clinical research workforce, especially at the physician/principal investigator level. Participants discussed the "failure of medical education to significantly increase the diversity [of the] physician workforce in the United States," Galson said.

Envisioning and Effecting Systemic Change

- There is optimism that change is possible and already taking place. "Now, like never before, this issue has risen to the top, not just within the medical research community, but within the public discourse at large," Krofah said.
- A systemic, enterprise-level, cooperative approach is needed to improve inclusivity in clinical trials, Galson reported, rather than the many disparate efforts by individual organizations that are currently occurring. There are models to scale and best practices to be shared, Krofah added. The clinical trials enterprise needs to move beyond "islands of excellence" to "a whole ecosystem of excellence for all people," she said.
- How to effect change was a topic across breakout group discussions, including the roles of mandates and enforcement, incentives, investments and capacity building, accountability, and the will to make change. More discussion is needed on the role of FDA in advancing inclusiveness in clinical trials, Galson suggested, such as the extent to which the agency has the authority to mandate changes.
- Learning from the ongoing response to the COVID-19 pandemic was a recurring topic of discussion. For example, Krofah asked, how can the infrastructure, networks, and collaborations be sustained and expanded to address other disease conditions that disproportionately affect particular communities?

4

Practical Applications for Technology to Enhance the Clinical Trials Enterprise

> **Highlights of Key Points Made by Individual Speakers**
>
> - The technology needed to drive change in the clinical trials enterprise already exists. What is lacking is coordination and an understanding of how to effectively use that technology to advance clinical trials. (Hirsch)
> - Technology can help inform patients about clinical trials and reduce the burden of participation, but it is not a silver-bullet solution for engaging more people in research. (Hastings)
> - The bidirectional flow of data can provide direct benefits to patients. "People are much more willing to give their data when they have the feeling that they are getting something out of it." (Brönneke)
> - Many of the tools, technologies, and processes that were implemented during the COVID-19 pandemic response could be adopted more broadly across the clinical trials enterprise, but not all will be sustainable outside of a crisis response. (Chang)
> - Data are needed to characterize the performance of technology-enabled, decentralized clinical trials based on parameters such as participant safety, participant and site experience, data privacy, and data integrity. (Tenaerts)
> - For greater integration of research and care, overlap is needed in the regulatory oversight of some of these areas. (Perakslis)

- Each interaction a patient has with the health system is an opportunity to foster trust in clinical trials and identify potential areas of hidden bias or inaccessibility in these encounters. (Roosz)
- Patients using digital health technologies should be able to trust that their information is secure. A holistic approach to data governance should balance data security with usability of the technology and include non-discrimination protections. (Coravos)

This segment of the four-part workshop focused on practical applications of technology to transform the clinical trials enterprise for 2030. Participants considered ways that thoughtful and deliberate use of digital technologies could support the goals of improving person-centeredness and inclusivity of clinical trials and ensuring resilience, sustainability, and transparency in the clinical trials enterprise.

THE ROAD TO 2030: PERSPECTIVES FROM THE FIELD

Frontline Experience: A Panel Discussion

In this session, three panelists described how they are working to apply technology practically in pursuit of an improved clinical trials enterprise. Panelists included Tara Hastings, senior associate director for Patient Engagement at The Michael J. Fox Foundation for Parkinson's Research; Jan Benedikt Brönneke, director, Law and Economics of Health Technologies at the health innovation hub (hih) of the German Federal Ministry of Health; and Bradford Hirsch, chief executive officer (CEO) of SignalPath Research. To open the session, Jennifer Goldsack, executive director of the Digital Medicine Society and session moderator, said that an enhanced clinical trials enterprise for the future does not necessarily require more technology, but, rather, more solved problems. Current and emerging technologies are "tools in the toolbox" that can help drive the enterprise to become safer, more effective, more efficient, and more equitable.

"Tools in the Toolbox"

Hirsch stated that the technology needed to drive change in the clinical trials enterprise already exists. What is lacking is coordination and an understanding of how to effectively use that technology to advance clinical trials. For example, he said stakeholders may not be familiar with currently available operational technology for clinical trial sites (e.g., tools for regulatory document management, operational management for trials, and payment infrastructure). There is an opportunity to bring together different technology products to integrate the generation of clinical trial data and collection of real-world data, he said, while preserving essential patient–clinician relationships.

Hastings added that technology can help inform patients on clinical trial participation. Technology can also be deployed to help reduce the burden of trial participation, especially for patients with progressive disorders, such as Parkinson's disease (e.g., by reducing the number of in-person visits required). She noted, however, that technology is not a silver-bullet solution for engaging more people in research. Studies funded by The Michael J. Fox Foundation for Parkinson's Research have found that barriers to participation include time, acceptability, and language barriers, but also access to technology. This means it is important to find ways to be inclusive and to connect with those in the community who may not have wireless Internet access or the ability to use it, for example.

Bidirectional Information Flow

Hastings pointed out that technology is "a two-way street." It is not just about what trial participants may contribute to research, but also what the clinical trials enterprise can give back to participants and their providers that could better inform their own health care and choices. The bidirectional flow of information can help enable more productive conversations between patients and their providers and offer patients more insight into their own care, she said.

As Germany has been implementing the use of digital health technologies to enhance the delivery of health care following the passage of the Digital Health Care Act in 2019,[1] it has become clear that there are opportunities to use these tools for clinical evidence generation as well, Brönneke said. However, patients in Germany have expressed concern that their data could be misused. The European Union General Data Protection Regulation (GDPR) addresses data privacy, including the use of patient data and the sharing of data for purposes other than those originally intended. While implementation of the GDPR promotes trust among patients, Brönneke described the regulation as restrictive to the point of reducing the potential benefits that could be derived from the data.

As mentioned above, the bidirectional flow of data can provide direct benefits to patients, and Brönneke observed that "people are much more

---

[1] For more information about the law, see a summary written by hih at https://hih-2025.de/dvg-a-summary-of-germanys-new-law-for-digital-health-applications (accessed August 3, 2021).

willing to give their data when they have the feeling that they are getting something out of it." For example, he noted that many people freely share personal information on social media because they feel they receive something of value in return. Similarly, patients are more likely to share their health data when they feel included in the clinical research process. As an example, Brönneke mentioned the digital health applications process in Germany. This process allows for research use of the real-world data associated with digital therapeutics, and patients who share their data via an approved digital health application receive direct and timely feedback.

Coordination and Integration of Technical Solutions to Improve the Patient Experience

Hirsch shared his personal experience as a recent participant in a COVID-19 vaccine clinical trial, summarizing the experience as "a bit of a mess." What was intended to be an hour-long initial visit lasted more than 6 hours. This was due, he said, to a lack of coordination across the multiple technology elements from five different vendors that were being used for the trial (e.g., the eConsent platform, the app for receiving payment for participation, the app for reporting symptoms). He suggested that the challenge was not the technology itself, but rather the lack of coordination. Technologies used for a trial should be coordinated in advance and deployed in a way that focuses on the user experience, educating trial participants and engaging them in the process.

Technology solutions are siloed, in part, because they are expensive and complex to develop, Hirsch said. Solutions must correctly follow data privacy and security regulations to protect patient information and the integrity of trial data. What is needed, Hirsch said, is agreement among regulatory agencies on what policies and oversight are necessary to govern and coordinate use of digital health technologies in clinical trials, such that relevant policies are streamlined and more easily understood by developers working in different areas. In addition, he said, there is a need for better coordination among technology developers and other stakeholders working within those defined policies. Developers are not opposed to eliminating the siloes, he said, but there must be investment in infrastructures that can support and facilitate alignment.

Brönneke suggested that responsibility for coordination falls primarily on the technology developers, but he added that more encouraging regulatory policies would have a positive impact. He observed that siloed data are barriers to coordination. In Germany, the health care system is encouraged to increase the interoperability of health data by using Fast Healthcare Interoperability Resources profiles and the internationally standardized SNOMED CT terminology[2] for recording clinical information.[3] He noted that regulatory acceptance of real-world evidence varies by country and remains limited in some places, and suggested that regulatory frameworks could include broader definitions of acceptable clinical trials (e.g., prospective cohort studies).

Hastings emphasized the need for co-development of clinical trial technologies with the people the products are intended to serve. As an example, she said that a wearable device, such as a watch, can be useful for many people, but people with Parkinson's disease often have difficulty managing the watchband, and the watch can snag on clothing during tremors. In addition, she said that "sponsors have the opportunity to work with patients to understand how technology actually get[s] integrated." She suggested that walking a patient through a mock study visit could help identify challenges and areas where technology might be able to improve the participant experience. Hastings noted that it is challenging to measure the return on investment of patient involvement in drug development, and it can therefore be difficult to justify extending project time lines to allow for gathering patient input. She suggested that stakeholders work collectively to identify potential measures and to educate investors about both the value of designing technology up front to meet patient needs and the risks of not doing so. Her vision for 2030 is that study participants would not have to manage many different technology elements (e.g., a watch, an app) to achieve the same outcome. Uncoordinated technology elements can also create confusion for regulators and payers, she noted. Hastings said the patient community is ready and willing to contribute to finding solutions and that advocacy groups can play a role by serving as precompetitive conveners.

A unified trial experience for patients should include technology elements that flow together, and coordination of technology across the clinical site experience to ensure that trials are efficiently executed and necessary datasets are obtained, Hirsch summarized. The architecture to support integration across technology products exists, he said, but regulatory policies must be coordinated. Thinking intentionally about the patient experience and the site experience "cascades into a better experience for participants, higher accessibility, and generation of higher quality, more accessible data," Goldsack concluded.

---

[2] For more information on SNOMED, see https://www.snomed.org (accessed July 26, 2021).

[3] For more information on the SNOMED CT policy adopted by the German Federal Institute for Drugs and Medical Devices, see https://www.bfarm.de/EN/Code-systems/Terminologies/SNOMED-CT/_node.html (accessed August 3, 2021).

THE ROAD TO 2030: VISIONS OF WHAT IS POSSIBLE

Speakers in this session provided examples of collaboration and innovation toward implementing digital technologies in clinical trials. Janice Chang, chief operating officer at TransCelerate, discussed some of the lessons learned from the response by TransCelerate member companies to the COVID-19 pandemic and shared her perspective on the role of technology in moving toward 2030. Pamela Tenaerts, chief scientific officer at Medable and former executive director at CTTI, discussed implementing technology to enable decentralized clinical trials in a responsible way. The session was moderated by Anita Allen, professor of law and philosophy at the University of Pennsylvania Carey Law School.

Collaboration in Action: The TransCelerate COVID-19 Response

TransCelerate is a global not-for-profit entity that serves as a catalyst for industry-wide collaboration, Chang said. More than 1,000 experts from 20 member companies are working together on more than 30 projects that align with TransCelerate's three strategic priorities: (1) harmonize process and share information; (2) improve the patient and site experience; and (3) enhance sponsor efficiencies and drug safety.[4] Chang emphasized that TransCelerate works diligently and proactively to ensure that different stakeholder groups are engaged in these projects, including regulatory authorities, clinical sites, CROs, technology vendors, and others.

Pandemic Response

Since the early days of the COVID-19 pandemic, Chang said there has been an "unparalleled willingness" by TransCelerate member companies to share, learn from each other, and collaborate to identify solutions for maintaining trial continuity during the pandemic. Product sponsors deployed a range of novel and non-traditional technologies, tools, and methods in a crisis-response environment. Practical solutions launched by TransCelerate included, for example, a COVID-19 data-sharing module in TransCelerate's existing DataCelerate platform and a protocol deviation toolkit, which she said are available not just to member companies, but to any qualified stakeholders.

Chang highlighted some of the considerations when implementing novel, non-traditional continuity tools and technologies during a crisis. For example, it is important to ensure that tools and technologies intended

---

[4] For more information about TransCelerate, see https://www.transceleratebiopharmainc.com (accessed July 1, 2021).

to reduce the burden on participants do not inadvertently increase the burden on sites, and vice versa. Additionally, stakeholders should consider how tools and technologies are delivered to patients and sites and how training can be effectively deployed in a virtual setting. She added that it is critical to ensure that data integrity and privacy are not compromised when implementing new tools and technologies for data collection. She referred participants to the TransCelerate website for information on these and other resources, including a paper sharing best practices and assessing how the lessons learned from the COVID-19 response could inform modernization of the clinical trials enterprise after the pandemic.[5] Stakeholders in the clinical trials ecosystem now have an opportunity to create lasting change by shifting to a collaborative mindset, she said. She closed by paraphrasing a popular adage: "To change fast, go alone. To go far, we have to go together."

Reprioritizing for the Future

Responding to the COVID-19 pandemic in an agile manner presented TransCelerate with opportunities to evolve and to reprioritize its collaborative initiatives around two main themes. The first theme, modernization, involves incorporating new and innovative technologies and processes that simplify and improve participant experiences while ensuring that participant safety and data reliability are maintained, Chang explained. The second theme centers around enabling a more dynamic data ecosystem to amplify the power of the vast amounts of data being generated and accelerate product development. Initiatives are focused on data usage, versatility, and accessibility.

Chang observed that, compared with other industries, the clinical trials enterprise is "a little stuck when it comes to … adopting innovative technologies," and said the industry has "an obligation to … evolve the way we conduct our research and development activities." She emphasized the need to thoughtfully consider which tools, technologies, and processes implemented during the COVID-19 pandemic response could be adopted more broadly across the clinical trials enterprise, noting that not all will be sustainable outside of a crisis response.

Technology-Enabled Decentralized Clinical Trials

Tenaerts asserted that "We need to improve our evidence-generating system so that we can answer more questions about what will impact

---

[5] See https://www.transceleratebiopharmainc.com/initiatives/modernizing-clinical-trial-conduct (accessed July 1, 2021).

health." Medable is working to enable decentralized clinical trials thorough appropriate and responsible use of technology.[6] Decentralized clinical trials are still clinical trials, Tenaerts said, and should (1) ensure participant safety and patient-centricity; (2) deliver reliable, actionable data to decision makers, including care providers, patients, and regulatory agencies; and (3) improve participant and site satisfaction with the clinical trial process. Several individual workshop participants, including Robert Califf of Verily Life Sciences (see Chapter 2) and breakout participants summarized in Chapter 3, emphasized that the practical application of digital health technologies can improve access to clinical trials for participants who may not live near traditional brick-and-mortar clinical trial sites.

Drawing on her prior experience at CTTI, Tenaerts emphasized the importance of engaging all stakeholders in clinical trials when seeking solutions to difficult problems. In developing clinical trial solutions for decentralized trials, she said that Medable has included experts in product design and technology as partners in the discussions. Although these stakeholders might not have extensive clinical trials experience, they bring a different perspective and can help formulate new approaches to address persistent problems, she said.

Tenaerts highlighted the following three main areas where technology-enabled decentralized clinical trials can face barriers to adoption and implementation:

- **Regulatory.** A key consideration for implementing new technologies in clinical trials is whether such changes to methodology will meet regulatory requirements, Tenaerts said. Acceptability might also vary depending on the country and agency.
- **Legal.** There are a host of potential legal considerations when implementing new technologies in clinical trials. For example, state licensing boards have different requirements for the practice of telemedicine. Although some licensing requirements were temporarily suspended during the COVID-19 pandemic response, Tenaerts observed that many are being reinstated as the pandemic continues. Authentication of users can be challenging when appointments or interactions are not done in person and involve parties without an established provider–patient relationship, and laws dealing with authentication practices such as electronic signatures vary by country.
- **Practical.** A key practical consideration for implementing innovative technologies in clinical trials is building trust in the new

---

[6] For more information about Medable, see https://www.medable.com (accessed July 1, 2021).

systems, Tenaerts said. She also pointed out that just because something can be done does not mean it should be done. Using decentralized methods can lead to "loss of human connection," and she said it might be better to retain some in-person encounters by using local laboratories and imaging centers, or arranging for local nurses to visit trial participants' homes. Basic human nature can also be a hurdle, and changing behavior can be difficult. Studies in behavioral economics show that people often choose the perceived easiest option to avoid having to make a complex decision, and focus on the immediate returns rather than longer term implications of their decisions. Professional hesitancy is also a barrier, she said, as there are often concerns that poor trial outcomes might be blamed on the use of the new methodology.

To overcome these hurdles, Tenaerts said the clinical trials community needs to generate data that characterize the performance of technology-enabled decentralized clinical trials. This includes evidence demonstrating how technology helps to keep trial participants safe with regard to both potential adverse events, and data privacy and security concerns. It is also important to demonstrate that conducting technology-enabled decentralized trials does not adversely affect the clinical trial data in any way. For example, evidence is needed to demonstrate that enrollment is representative and inclusive, and that the resulting clinical trial data are actionable and reliable. Tenaerts pointed out that the use of technology can potentially improve the data collection process, but without caution and careful monitoring can also introduce systematic bias or error. Data are also needed that demonstrate how conducting technology-enabled decentralized trials leads to a better trial experience for both participants and sites, and enhances trust in the clinical trials enterprise.

Tenaerts noted that some trials conducted during the COVID-19 pandemic were decentralized out of necessity (i.e., they were deemed to be critical trials, and decentralization was necessary to keep the trials going). The question, she said, is how to build on this base of experience and expand the use of decentralized trials. She noted that the FDA Oncology Center of Excellence is now requesting that data collected remotely be specifically tagged in an effort to better understand the impact of decentralizing trials (e.g., How does decentralization impact the rates of missed visits and missing data? What is the impact of remote administration of the investigational product on compliance?).

Short-Term Goals for Applying Technology to Simplify Clinical Trials and Improve the Patient Experience: Panel and Breakout Discussion Highlights

Following the panel discussion, online participants were divided into virtual Zoom breakout rooms to consider how technology might be applied toward achieving the vision of the 2030 clinical trials enterprise. In this breakout session, groups focused on two goals: enabling a more person-centered and easily accessible clinical trials enterprise; and simplifying trials (e.g., less active data collection, fewer site visits, reduced costs) while still generating high-quality data and robust answers to relevant clinical questions. Participants discussed practical applications of technologies, barriers to implementation and use, and where and by whom these technologies would be used relative to these goals. Upon reconvening in plenary session, Goldsack briefly reflected on the panel and breakout group discussions.

Participants discussed how to engage with target populations "thoughtfully, deliberately, using technology as a new tool in the toolbox, with eyes on patient safety and getting the best data that we can," Goldsack summarized. Comments addressed ways in which the use of technologies could lead to greater success in implementing concepts such as inclusivity by design and taking a person-centric approach. It was pointed out, Goldsack relayed, that clinical trial workflows will evolve as technologies are implemented, and they might look different from today's workflows, perhaps with different actors and occurring in different places (e.g., pop-up clinics for vaccinations). She added that thinking about change management and new ways of working is as essential to success as implementing new technologies. Goldsack and Amy Abernethy, former principal deputy commissioner for food and drugs at FDA, discussed taking a "product mindset" when building and deploying technologies for the future clinical trials enterprise. Examples are developing modules that could be coordinated and integrated, and creating minimal viable products for user feedback. In doing so, Goldsack explained, "we are able to deliver to the target user a product that is inherently valuable and inherently appealing."

Long-Term Goals for Applying Technology to Improve Trial Diversity and Inclusivity: Panel and Breakout Discussion Highlights

In this breakout session, groups focused on the role of technology in achieving the goal of establishing a clinical trials enterprise that is more diverse, equitable, and inclusive, and the goal of establishing a national network of community-based clinical trial sites. Participants discussed practical applications of technologies, barriers to implementation and use, and where and by whom these technologies would be used relative to these goals. Upon reconvening in plenary session, Allen briefly reflected on the panel and breakout group discussions.

As discussed throughout the panels and breakout groups, "we need to find ways to connect to underserved communities," Allen summarized. This includes more community-based programming and workforce training, for example. In developing clinical research training opportunities for the clinicians and staff in underserved communities, participants discussed that the clinical research enterprise needs to learn first from them about their training needs and resource challenges. It was pointed out that simply implementing technologies to decentralize trials will not solve all the challenges these community clinicians are facing.

Another topic of discussion, Allen noted, was the importance of developing culturally competent approaches to implementing new technologies. Different communities and cultures access and use technology differently, and failure to understand this could exacerbate health disparities. It was also noted that there are many variations within a given broad population or cultural group, and there is a need to understand local context (e.g., the five main Census categories for race are composed of many different cultures). Discussion also continued on need to build trust in the clinical research enterprise and clinical trials.

Finally, participants discussed who in the clinical trials ecosystem is responsible for implementing the technology changes that could advance the diversity and inclusiveness of clinical trials. "It is a broad participation of all the stakeholders," Allen summarized, including government, regulators, patients, clinicians, and others.

REFLECTIONS ON REALIZING THE POTENTIAL OF TECHNOLOGY IN CLINICAL TRIALS

Andy Coravos, co-founder and CEO of Elektra Labs (renamed Human-First since the time of the workshop); Eric Perakslis, chief science and digital officer at the Duke Clinical Research Institute; and Sam Roosz, co-founder and CEO of Crescendo Health reflected on realizing the vision of a transformed clinical trials enterprise through the thoughtful and responsible deployment of technologies. The discussion drew from an associated *Health Affairs* blog post in which they envision how the lives of four fictional individuals could be changed with the integration of technologies into the clinical trials enterprise.[7] The discussion was moderated by Esther Krofah.

---

[7] This discussion is based on a blog post titled *The Future of Clinical Trials: How Will New Technologies Affect the Lives of Participants?*, available at https://www.healthaffairs.org/do/10.1377/hblog20210505.673654/full (accessed July 1, 2021).

Applying Digital Health Technology in Clinical Trials

Krofah and Roosz noted that a recurring theme during this part of the workshop was that, in some cases, clinical trial conduct and trial participant experience could be improved through the practical use of existing digital health technologies. Panelists discussed some of the considerations for stakeholders seeking to better integrate digital health technologies into clinical trials.[8]

Recognizing that the time is now and acknowledge that these technology approaches are implementable. Roosz said there is an opportunity to move quickly to selectively implement new technologies in appropriate clinical trials that can help deliver meaningful products to patients. "We do not need to build all these new technologies," he said. "We already have them sitting at our fingertips." He called on participants to "suspend disbelief about what is possible" and break the habit of meeting any new proposal with counterarguments about why they should not be tried. Start from the position that implementation of a particular technology to advance a specific clinical trial is achievable, and then work to address the logistical and institutional challenges.

Focusing on collaboration, inclusion, and trust. Reflecting on his career in technology, Perakslis said "the technology has not been the hard part. It is collaboration. It is trust. It is listening that tends to be difficult." He agreed there are digital health technologies already available and said the focus should not be on developing another app, data network, or database. The focus should be on fostering cooperation and promoting inclusion and trust, and he emphasized the importance of working with existing networks of doctors and community health workers. Roosz agreed and said trust is the core of any relationship between a patient and a care provider, whether as part of routine clinical care or in the context of a clinical trial. He suggested that each time a patient interacts with the health system, it is an opportunity to foster trust in clinical trials, and identify potential areas of hidden bias or inaccessibility in these encounters. He added that engagement of people in their communities ("on their turf"), by providers who look like them and speak their languages, is one key way to start building trust.

Taking a holistic approach to data governance. Although much attention is given to issues of data privacy, Coravos suggested that it is more important to talk about data governance—who gets access to what data and when. Patients should be able to trust that their information is secure

---

[8] Coravos also referred participants to *The Playbook*, a guide for developing and deploying digital clinical measures in clinical trials, health care, and public health developed by the Digital Medicine Society. See https://playbook.dimesociety.org (accessed July 1, 2021).

when they use digital health technologies, and there is ongoing discussion about how to balance data security with usability of the technology. She emphasized that a holistic approach to governance of health data should include non-discrimination protections for patients. Roosz noted that other elements of good data governance including transparency of how data are handled, and consent from patients for how their data are used. Reporting information back to trial participants is important, he said, "so that they, as a contributor and a partner in this clinical trials enterprise, are able to celebrate with the investigators the results and learnings from that study."

Meeting people where they are. When designing a clinical trial, start with an understanding of what measures and outcomes matter to patients, Coravos said. Then determine if technology provides solutions participants want. Coravos suggested that patient-centeredness is about making sure the patient has choices. Do not make assumptions about what patients do or do not want, she said. For example, some patients might not want to draw their own blood sample, even if the technology to do so is available. Some people might prefer more support when collecting and providing their data in a trial.

Better integrating the practice of medicine and the development of medical products. There are gaps in knowledge between experts who specialize in developing medical products and practicing clinicians. "To move clinical trials into the community, we have to create the right type of overlap so that we ... have more fluency between research and care," Perakslis said. As an example of potential overlap, he noted the similarities between a clinical trial case report form and the EHR entries for a clinical care visit, but emphasized only the information in the case report form is included in a clinical trial while the natural history collected in the EHR is often lost. He advocated for considering how providers could better use patient care interactions as opportunities to engage people in clinical research, and using technologies to make the integration more seamless for patients and providers.

Potential Next-Step Actions for Stakeholders

Krofah asked panelists to suggest next-step actions by stakeholders in the clinical trials enterprise to begin implementing technologies toward their vision for 2030 now. They suggested the following actions:

- **Modeling what has worked in other venues.** Perakslis mentioned hospice care as an example of a successful "click and mortar" business model (i.e., one that functions both online and in person). Hospice is a domain of care that rapidly moves a person from clinical care to personalized care at home or in a dedicated facility. He proposed that moving a person into a clinical trial directly from a care encounter could happen in a similar manner. For example, an individual could be referred for a trial, then trial staff could conduct a home visit, using digital technologies for collecting and moving data. This approach, deploying both humans and technology, could be a good first step as the system evolves toward decentralized trials.

- **Actively participating in process of policy making and rule making.** Coravos pointed out that proposed rules and regulations are posted for public comment, and regulators are required to review all comments submitted. She described this as a powerful way for individuals to contribute to the policy-making process. Social media posts and online discussions may be widely read or viewed, but comments submitted to regulators during open comment periods directly inform policy decisions. Roosz agreed and encouraged participants to take opportunities to submit comments as stakeholders by profession and as individuals. Coravos noted that there are opportunities for collaboration to help develop prototypes for rules that have not yet been written, and to test them in different settings. "Make the change that we would like to see," she said.
- **Picking one technology solution and taking the first step.** Roosz emphasized that the problems with integrating and scaling new technologies in clinical trials do not need to be solved all at once. He encouraged those who are conducting studies to choose one or several new methodologies, use them, and solicit feedback from stakeholders on how they impacted the conduct of the trial and the patient experience. "We might be surprised with the quality that these new approaches actually bring to what have been pretty unchanging methods in the past," he said.

5

Building a More Resilient, Sustainable, and Transparent Clinical Trials Enterprise

> **Highlights of Key Points Made by Individual Speakers**
>
> - "Clinical trial[s are] part of good quality clinical care; they are not an optional extra." (Landray)
> - For the clinical trials enterprise to be sustainable, it has to be worthwhile and practical for frontline health care providers who care for underrepresented populations to participate as investigators. (Ofili)
> - Sustainability of the clinical trials enterprise requires informing the public about trials, listening to patients, and dispelling myths about the willingness of diverse populations to participate in trials. (Segarra-Vázquez)
> - A fresh, unencumbered perspective combined with the purposeful use of existing resources and networks are both needed to build out a community-based clinical research infrastructure. (Lewis-Hall)
> - Developing a person-centered communication approach requires an understanding of what trust and transparency mean to different people. (Southwell)
> - People's relationships outside of the formal health care system, including family, friends, coworkers, classmates, and others with whom they have trusted relationships, most influence their health-related decisions and habits they adopt. (Bryson)

> - Simply issuing recommendations is not sufficient to change behavior. Providing operational tools can aid stakeholders in implementing policy and practice recommendations to improve clinical trials. (Tenaerts)

The focus of this segment of the four-part workshop was on the elements needed to build a more resilient, sustainable, and transparent clinical trials enterprise by 2030. Participants discussed the need for convergence and integration of clinical research and clinical practice; data sharing and management; and more efficient, engaging scientific communication.

THE ROAD TO 2030: PERSPECTIVES FROM THE FIELD

Martin Landray, professor of medicine and epidemiology at the Nuffield Department of Population Health at the University of Oxford, discussed the Randomized Evaluation of COVID-19 Therapy (RECOVERY) Trial as an example to highlight the importance of conducting randomized clinical trials and demonstrate how clinical trials can be a core component of clinical care. Three panelists then shared their frontline experience addressing some of the challenges facing the clinical trials enterprise.

The "Magic" of Randomization: The RECOVERY Trial Experience

In response to the significant mortality associated with COVID-19, hundreds of different treatments were being tried in practice. There were many opinions about the value of these treatments, often based on small, inconclusive randomized trials, uncontrolled case series, and theoretical work, but reliable data supporting the use of these treatments was not available, Landray said. RECOVERY[1] was designed to evaluate the efficacy of a range of interventions repurposed to treat individuals hospitalized with COVID-19 in the United Kingdom. For COVID-19, as for many other diseases, Landray said finding a single treatment that quickly cures all patients is unlikely, and large-scale randomization is required to identify effective treatments that offer modest improvements in outcomes of importance (e.g., reduced mortality).

---

[1] ClinicalTrials.gov Identifier: NCT04381936. See also https://www.recoverytrial.net (accessed July 1, 2021).

Design of the RECOVERY Trial

Three key principles were embedded within the design of RECOVERY: (1) to obtain robust results that can rapidly impact care; (2) to consider the well-being of the patients; and (3) to consider the well-being of the staff, Landray explained. The study was designed to focus strictly on identifying products that could save lives, he said. The trial entailed randomization of the relevant populations and comprehensive follow-up, as well as communication, collaboration, and broad transparency (e.g., communication with researchers, the medical community, patients, the public). Landray referred workshop participants to a recent publication in which he describes how smart trial design and streamlined operations, integrated data and technology, and flexible regulatory approaches can lead to improved patient care and public health (Collins et al., 2020).

These principles were put into practice for the launch of RECOVERY in March 2020. The relevant population to be randomized was patients who were hospitalized and believed to have COVID-19 (see Figure 5-1). Enrollment in RECOVERY was open to anyone admitted to any hospital in the United Kingdom, which Landray said enhanced diversity and inclusivity. "You cannot recruit people from diverse communities if you

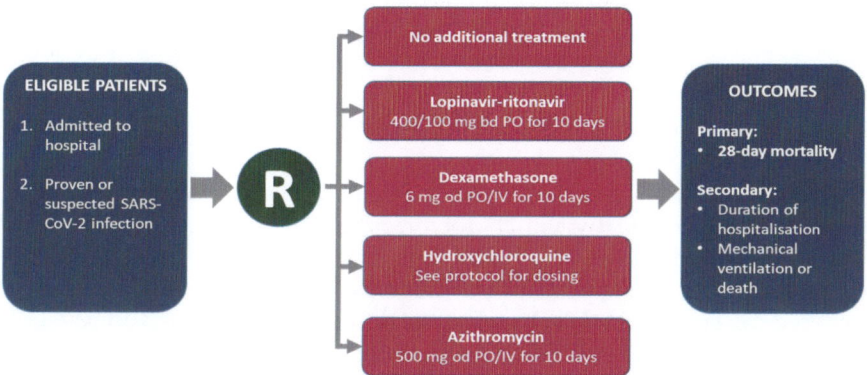

FIGURE 5-1 Basic protocol design for the first phase of the RECOVERY trial.
NOTES: Exclusion criteria were applied prior to randomization (e.g., if there was a contraindication for the participant to receive a particular intervention, that treatment arm would be removed as an option before randomization of that participant, which Landray said provides for an unbiased assessment of the treatments). The protocol was subsequently adapted to include multiple, factorial randomization.
NOTE: R = randomization; SARS-CoV-2 = severe acute respiratory syndrome coronavirus 2.
SOURCE: Landray presentation, March 24, 2021.

don't locate the studies in diverse locations," he said. As a result of the simplified recruitment, enrollment, and consent processes, more than 10,000 participants were enrolled during the first 8 weeks of the study. RECOVERY continues to enroll, and Landray noted that 20,000 participants were enrolled from December 2020 through February 2021.

The primary outcome for RECOVERY was mortality. Follow-up was facilitated using a one-page, online case report form and supplemented by linkage to existing UK National Health Service (NHS) datasets on hospitalization, mortality, primary care, critical care, specific diseases, and COVID-19. Leveraging existing information reduces workload for the trialists and facilitates long-term follow-up, Landray explained. He noted that, although NHS is the primary provider of health care in the United Kingdom, data are collected in many different databases as NHS spans 4 nations, nearly 200 acute hospital organizations, and 10,000 primary care practices. As an example, he said that six different datasets were accessed for information about mortality for the primary outcome. The associated data integration challenges were significant, but worthwhile to obtain more robust information, he said.

Results from RECOVERY

Landray briefly described some of the results from RECOVERY thus far. He shared, for example, that hydroxychloroquine, lopinavir–ritonavir, and azithromycin were not shown to have a clinically meaningful benefit for hospitalized COVID-19 patients, despite having been widely recommended, promoted, and used by clinicians in the United States and many other parts of the world.

By contrast, although the use of dexamethasone was considered to be contraindicated by many doctors, the clear and compelling data from RECOVERY showed that it reduced mortality in those patients who required oxygen or ventilation. As evidence of the impact of sufficiently powered randomized trials, Landray said these results were publicized at lunchtime on June 16, 2020, and by teatime, dexamethasone treatment of hospitalized COVID-19 patients who needed oxygen or ventilation was national policy in every UK hospital.[2] Other nations followed suit and it had been estimated that, at the time of the workshop, at least 600,000 lives had been saved as a result of this policy change.

As another example, Landray showed how data from RECOVERY provided clear results regarding the ability of the anti-inflammatory drug tocilizumab to reduce mortality for some COVID-19 patients with

---

[2] See https://www.nejm.org/doi/10.1056/NEJMoa2021436 (accessed February 14, 2022).

hypoxia and inflammation, after numerous prior small studies were inconclusive.

Lessons from RECOVERY

Beyond the clinical findings, RECOVERY demonstrates how randomized trials can be a core component of quality clinical care. RECOVERY was embedded within existing hospital processes and procedures, Landray said, and on average about 10 percent of patients admitted with COVID-19 across NHS hospitals were enrolled in the trial. In addition, he discussed six takeaway lessons from RECOVERY (see Box 5-1) and said that involvement with the trial has inspired more junior doctors to want to become active in clinical research.

"Clinical trial[s are] part of good quality clinical care; they are not an optional extra," Landray said. He emphasized that the "arbitrary use of unproven treatments is a disservice to patient care and public health," raising false hopes, wasting resources, and missing opportunities to learn and improve care.

In closing, Landray reiterated that trials need to be feasible for trial participants and staff, inclusive, and focused on outcomes of importance to patients. Transforming to a system in which trials are part of care

---

BOX 5-1
Lessons from RECOVERY

Martin Landray, professor of medicine and epidemiology at the Nuffield Department of Population Health at the University of Oxford, highlighted six key elements of success for the RECOVERY trials in the United Kingdom that could be applied to clinical trials in the United States.

- The RECOVERY trials are designed to allow easy participation.
- The RECOVERY protocol was quickly approved at the national level and adopted by all hospitals in Britain.
- Background patient data provided by the UK National Health Service helped to simplify the research process.
- Support from leaders in government health care ensured widespread cooperation by hospitals.
- Britain has a national system of research nurses who were rapidly redeployed to work on COVID-19 research.
- The British effort was incorporated as part of everyday clinical care in hospitals.

SOURCES: Landray presentation, March 24, 2021; Emanuel et al., 2020.

requires leadership, coordination, fairness, and transparency, and creation of a culture in which clinical research is for everyone—including participants and frontline medical staff.

Frontline Experience: A Panel Discussion

Elizabeth Ofili, contact principal investigator at the Research Centers in Minority Institutions Coordinating Center, shared her perspective as a physician on integrating clinical care and clinical research to promote inclusivity and enhance the quality of care. Bárbara Segarra-Vázquez, dean of the School of Health Professions at the University of Puerto Rico, shared her perspective as a patient on what is needed to sustain the clinical trials enterprise. Freda Lewis-Hall, former senior medical advisor at Pfizer Inc. (retired), drew on her career experience in the pharmaceutical industry as she discussed building out the community-based clinical research infrastructure. The session was moderated by Chris Austin, director of the National Center for Advancing Translational Sciences (NCATS) at NIH.

Integrating Care and Research to Promote Inclusivity

The current clinical trials model is centered in academia, and there is a need to decentralize trials and engage the community and community practitioners. Until representation of certain populations and groups in trials is improved, it will be impossible to achieve health equity, Ofili said. For the clinical trials enterprise to be sustainable, it has to be worthwhile for frontline health care providers who care for predominantly underrepresented populations to participate as investigators. "Community providers are interested and want to participate," she said, but there are practical issues to be addressed. With an innovation award from NCATS, Ofili and colleagues are working directly with some of these practitioners to overcome critical barriers to inclusivity. One barrier is the inability during a brief patient encounter to extract data from their EHR that could enhance quality of care. Combining quality care and clinical research at the point of care requires investment, she said, and providers need training on how to use the technology and platforms to extract data. Ofili also highlighted the need for metrics to track progress as new provider groups become part of the clinical trials enterprise.

Engaging Patients in the Trial Process to Drive Sustainability

As an investigator and a two-time breast cancer survivor, Segarra-Vázquez has experience on both sides of clinical trials, and she said that sustainability of the enterprise requires informing the public about trials, listening to patients, and dispelling myths about the willingness of diverse populations to participate in trials.

"Knowledge is power," Segarra-Vázquez said, and the public should be informed about clinical trials so they are armed with the knowledge when the opportunity to participate arises. Patients are often approached about enrolling in a clinical trial when they have just been diagnosed with a disease, or even while being prepped for a procedure. They are focused on dealing with concerns and unknowns about their future, and most have little to no familiarity with clinical trials. Grasping the information about enrolling in a trial is even more challenging for those whose native language differs from that spoken by the trial staff, and she added that learning about a trial in an unfamiliar language does not instill trust in the enterprise. Just as people are constantly learning about products through commercials, social media, and the Internet, they should be constantly learning about clinical trials, Segarra-Vázquez said. She emphasized the power of storytelling to convey information about clinical trials.

It is a myth that Latinos and other minority groups do not want to participate in clinical trials, Segarra-Vázquez said. In her experience, people in Puerto Rico want to participate and the retention rate is high. However, minorities are often not told about trials or asked to participate. She also noted the importance of having a trial coordinator and other trial staff from traditionally underrepresented communities to interact with participants.

Patients are the experts in their own disease, and should be engaged in the trial process from the start, not as an afterthought, Segarra-Vázquez said. As a patient, "We can tell you what we want, how we want it, and how it will be successful," she said. It is especially important to ensure that diverse patients are included when collecting patient input. She noted that around 20 percent of cancer clinical trials fail to enroll as many patients as they need and close due to lack of recruitment (Korn et al., 2010). Listening to patients and "meeting the people where they are" to make trials more accessible can help to address this issue.

Envisioning and Achieving a Collaborative, Community-Based Clinical Research Infrastructure

Lewis-Hall observed that there is no master plan for transforming the clinical trials enterprise. Instead there are many different plans, and many people working "with great passion" who are making an impact, but there is no central action plan in which everyone can participate.

Drawing on her career experience in the pharmaceutical industry, Lewis-Hall suggested that a fresh, unencumbered perspective combined with the purposeful use of existing resources and networks are both needed to build out a community-based clinical research infrastructure. Starting with an unencumbered perspective, she asked, what does the structure of a clinical trials enterprise that can serve as the national evidence-generation platform look like? What incentives, regulations, and policies are needed to support those structures? What should the clinical trials workforce of the future look like? How can the clinical care environment participate in the collection of data to answer critical research questions in times of urgent need (e.g., during a pandemic), as well as ongoing questions of interest to patients, providers, and researchers to improve care?

At the same time, how can existing networks, such as the Patient-Centered Clinical Research Network, be coordinated to support this vision for the future? As an example, Lewis-Hall mentioned the Cancer Moonshot[3] approach to accelerating research, in which oncology networks are facilitating rapid, affordable oncology trials by using master protocols, platform trials, and other tools. In this regard, she said that the pharmaceutical industry is working to improve inclusion and productivity both through their actions as a collective of individual companies and through "meta-collaboration" with members of the communities the industry serves.

Overcoming Embedded Barriers to Collaboration

Austin pointed out that fundamental, curiosity-driven research forms the foundation of much of the research conducted in the United States. It is deeply embedded in an academic culture that has long rewarded individual ingenuity over the type of collaboration needed for the clinical trials enterprise envisioned for the future.

Ofili suggested that individual and institutional curiosity-driven research and collaborative, community-based research do not need to be mutually exclusive. The key is to identify "the right question to activate that curiosity" by partnering with those who know the disease or condition best, the patients, and their caregivers. Segarra-Vázquez added, "We have to train our young investigators to trust patients, talk to patients, and listen to patients." The interconnectedness of care and research, with the patient as a driver, will begin to decentralize and democratize clinical research, benefiting both the academic institutions and the community-based practices, Ofili said. Lewis-Hall agreed and said there is an opportunity to align goals and incentives by developing clear research questions with input from patients and caregivers, academia and industry, and the

---

[3] For more information, see https://www.cancer.gov/research/key-initiatives/moonshot-cancer-initiative (accessed August 3, 2021).

public. A practical action plan could begin with, for example, identifying the top 10 disparities in health outcomes to be addressed, the stakeholders who need to be at the table to address them, and the incentives that would inspire people to participate. Austin noted that empowering the community takes funding, and Ofili agreed that community providers involved in research need resources, guidance, and support. She added that, in her experience, community providers have innovative ideas for how to make the process of care more efficient.

THE ROAD TO 2030: VISIONS OF WHAT IS POSSIBLE

Brian Southwell, senior director of the Science in the Public Sphere Program at RTI International, discussed trust, transparency, and promoting public understanding of clinical trials. Dyan Bryson, founder and patient engagement strategist at Inspired Health Strategies, discussed facilitating the cultural change needed to support patient-centric and diverse clinical trials. Pamela Tenaerts shared insights on creating solutions and promoting trust and transparency. The session was moderated by Khair ElZarrad, deputy director of the Office of Medical Policy at FDA.

Embracing Person-Centered Communications About Clinical Trials[4]

A variety of factors can influence public understanding of drug research and development, Southwell said, including the salience of public information; the diffusion of misinformation; how information in the news is framed over time; existing understanding of science processes; and the state of science education. The vision of clinical trials for the future necessarily intersects with the public information environment.

Southwell described how a transformed clinical trials enterprise for 2030 might look.

- "Trials are advancing science by enrolling people who are the most directly impacted by and most directly burdened by diseases."
- Trial enrollment is at sufficient levels and people are less hesitant to participate.
- There are "partnerships [among] trial staff, media outlets, community-based organizations, and patients," and credible, locally relevant information is available to potential trial participants.

---

[4] This presentation is based on a blog post titled *A Future of Trusted Clinical Trials: Communication Strategies to Encourage Trust and Transparency*, available at https://www.healthaffairs.org/do/10.1377/hblog20210503.292254/full (accessed July 1, 2021).

- The results of trials are readily accessible to the public and are reported and celebrated in the media for contributing to community well-being.

There are crucial steps that must be taken to realize this vision, Southwell said, and resources will be needed to achieve the desired outcomes. A core element underlying this vision is person-centered communication about clinical trials. Developing a person-centered communication approach requires an understanding of what trust and transparency mean to different people, Southwell said.

Trust

From an academic perspective, trust is often associated with a perception of intellectual credibility or competence, Southwell said. Another popular and consequential dimension of trust is a perception of reliability or consistency (i.e., an expectation that an individual or institution will behave dependably or predictably). A related dimension of trust that is particularly relevant to clinical trials, Southwell explained, is trust as a perception of shared interest (also called encapsulated interest). In this sense, trust stems from the belief that others will act in your interest and to your benefit.

"If trust is rooted in both perception of shared interest and longstanding relationships," Southwell said, then investing in existing relationships and infrastructures would likely achieve better outcomes than launching new initiatives when, for example, working to increase diversity and inclusivity in clinical trials. In this example, trusted institutions might include the National Medical Association or Historically Black Colleges and Universities (HBCUs). Building trust between patients and the health care system can also help to counter the spread of misinformation, Southwell said.[5]

Transparency

Transparency is often thought of as simply making data and analyses available to others for their use. Research has shown, however, that simply making information (e.g., study results) available may not on its own guarantee public understanding, Southwell said.[6] Understanding

---

[5] Southwell referred participants to a blog post he authored for the ABIM Foundation titled *Trust as an Antidote to the Viral Spread of Medical Misinformation*, available at https://medium.com/@briansouthwell_94233/trust-as-an-antidote-to-the-viral-spread-of-medical-misinformation-12b0f2d3905a (accessed April 13, 2022).

[6] Southwell referred participants to a blog post he authored for the Medical Care Blog titled *Beyond Evidence Reporting: Evidence Translation in an Era of Uncertainty*, available at https://www.themedicalcareblog.com/evidence-translation (accessed July 1, 2021).

information about clinical trials is impacted by the general level of health and science literacy, but also by the public's ability to understand the concepts, vocabulary, acronyms, and statistics associated with research results. To facilitate transparency, Southwell said that researchers should take opportunities to translate their study data "in venues outside of peer-reviewed journals." As an example, he described how Michele Andrasik of the University of Washington discussed clinical trials for HIV vaccines on a public radio show (hosted by Southwell).[7] Andrasik told a "dramatic and compelling" story about how HIV vaccine research is conducted, which Southwell said lays groundwork for the public to understand and trust the clinical trials process and the results.

In closing, Southwell summarized three key steps needed for person-centered communication about clinical trials: "Acknowledge participant values, needs, and motivations" as they relate to participation in clinical trials; "build and maintain trust between researchers and participants by acknowledging shared interests"; and translate clinical trial methods and results to promote understanding and improve transparency of shared information.

Facilitating the Cultural Change Needed to Improve Trial Diversity

Envisioning the clinical trials enterprise for 2030, Bryson anticipated changes with regard to decentralizing clinical trials, the use of technology, and diversity in clinical trials. She focused her remarks on some of the changes needed to improve diversity in clinical trials, noting that decentralizing clinical trials can help to improve recruitment of diverse populations, and the use of technology for ongoing communication with trial participants can promote retention for existing trials and formation of positive long-term relationships that provide value to participants and potentially influence their decision to participate in future trials.

Bryson described three steps that clinical trial sponsors could take to improve the recruitment of diverse participants to clinical trials. She noted that these steps would be applied differently depending on the community.

- **Investing in building longitudinal relationships.** The prevalence of the disease or condition the investigational product is intended to treat will determine which communities and community-based organizations to engage, Bryson said. She emphasized the importance of investing in longitudinal relationships with the community in order to build trust.

---

[7] See https://measureradio.libsyn.com/encouraging-participation-in-clinical-trials (accessed July 1, 2021).

- **Building trust.** Bryson reiterated the point by Southwell that trust is a key element in successful recruitment of diverse participants for clinical trials. Consistency is important for maintaining trust, she said, and she advised trial sponsors to only commit to what they can deliver. Sponsors should also compensate partner organizations for the access they provide to the community and out of respect for their time spent in community engagement on behalf of the sponsor.
- **Coming to the community well before the recruitment is needed.** Speaking from her experience in industry, Bryson said that establishing community-based programs has consistently helped pharmaceutical companies to build long-term relationships that foster trust within the community. She emphasized the value of collaborating on existing efforts and the importance of putting in the time and work to build relationships well before attempting to recruit for a clinical trial (at least 6 months), and cautioned against "one-time only" events, which can damage credibility.

To emphasize the value of relationship building, Bryson said the average person spends only 67 minutes each year interacting with a health care provider. The rest of the time is spent interacting with their community, including family, friends, coworkers, classmates, and others with whom they have trusted relationships. These relationships outside of the formal health care system are the ones that most influence the health-related decisions people make and the habits they adopt.

Bryson referred participants to the work of author Glenna Crooks, who has mapped how an individual's decision making is influenced by the communities, or networks, with which they routinely interact (e.g., networks associated with their home/personal affairs, career, social life, spiritual life, family, and health/vitality).[8] Bryson shared Crooks's example of the influential networks for a hypothetical person, designated "Lucy" (see Figure 5-2). An estimated 71 of Lucy's connections will directly or indirectly influence a given decision. For example, Bryson explained, Lucy might consult five people directly about her decision, each of whom is influenced by other people in their own networks, and so on. This indicates that taking opportunities to raise awareness about participating in clinical trials among the people in Lucy's networks can ultimately influence Lucy's decision on whether she will choose to participate. To influence thinking or behavior, Bryson continued, "you don't have to always go directly to the person whose mind you want to change. You go to the people that they trust, [their] community."

---

[8] See https://glennacrooks.com (accessed July 1, 2021).

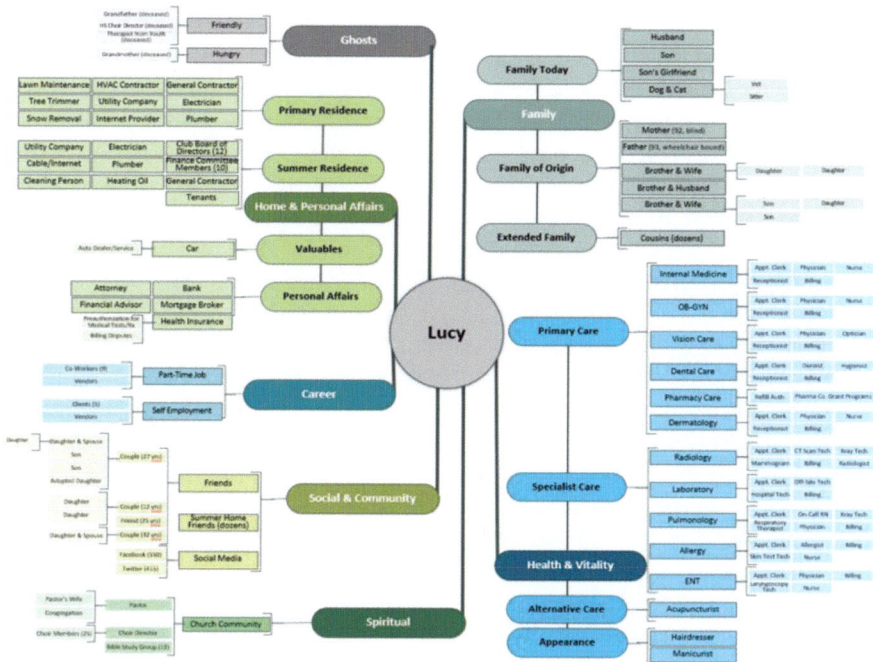

FIGURE 5-2 Complexity of community. Case example of the networks of influence for a hypothetical person, designated "Lucy."
SOURCES: Bryson presentation, March 24, 2021, and Glenna Crooks.

Creating Solutions That Promote Trust

Tenaerts described the approach taken by CTTI to promote a more sustainable and resilient clinical trials enterprise. CTTI aims to create structure and frameworks to support change, she said. As background, she referred participants to the Institute of Medicine workshop summary on envisioning the clinical trials enterprise for 2020 (IOM, 2012), and to CTTI's recently released vision statement on transforming clinical trials for 2030.[9]

A participatory, evidence-based approach to problem solving helps to build trust in the solutions developed, Tenaerts said. As a multi-stakeholder, public–private partnership, CTTI strives to be inclusive and give all stakeholders an equal voice in creating evidence-based solutions that will be relevant and have impact. Partners include clinical investi-

---

[9] See *Transforming Trials 2030*, available at https://ctti-clinicaltrials.org/who_we_are/transforming-trials-2030 (accessed April 13, 2022).

gators; patients, caregivers, and advocacy groups; academia; trade and professional organizations; IRBs; government and regulatory agencies; and industry. Tenaerts noted that CTTI is working to include data and technology companies as equal partners, rather than as vendors. To help enable an equal voice for patients, she said that the patient participants in their activities are reimbursed for their time away from work. Using quantitative and qualitative research methods, CTTI works to identify and understand issues and stakeholders' motivations and disincentives for change. CTTI then develops tools and recommendations to promote change and new norms. In the case of clinical trials, for example, a new norm would be including the patient voice from the beginning of the trial process. "Patients and patient advocates need to be included when the research questions are created, ... because they are the ones who ... are the experts on living with the disease," Tenaerts said.

One research method used by CTTI is the survey. Interestingly, a survey of CTTI members found that CTTI projects that had not yet issued recommendations had already begun to create change and have impact. Tenaerts reported that just being part of the project team and participating in the cross-stakeholder group discussions led to insights that inspired stakeholders to implement changes in the way they conduct their work. As a result, CTTI takes care to ensure diverse participation in projects and to allow for wider participation from different organizations. Tenaerts highlighted two general principles for CTTI projects. First, foster respect and collaboration among the project participants through open discussion. Second, recognize that these conversations can be difficult and there will be disagreement. "To maximize the benefit of collaboration you need to diverge before you converge," she said. In this regard, she said it is important to ensure that minority perspectives are heard, and to determine if those who have not contributed are simply in agreement or are not comfortable speaking up in the team setting.

One approach CTTI uses to develop recommendations is seeking to apply lessons learned from positive deviants. For a given area of interest, and under the same circumstances and constraints, there are isolated cases where applying innovative strategies has resulted in greater success (positive deviants). For example, Tenaerts said, CTTI will collect data to identify researchers who have been able to conduct a trial in a given health care setting when others have been less successful. These positive deviants are then engaged in CTTI's expert meetings and are interviewed in depth to identify themes underlying their success. This information is then used to develop and disseminate recommendations so that others can benefit (see Baxter et al., 2016).

Tenaerts said CTTI's experience has been that only issuing recommendations is not sufficient to change behavior. In 2013, CTTI began providing operational tools to aid stakeholders in implementing its policy and practice recommendations to improve clinical trials. In 2016, CTTI initiated activities designed to drive adoption of its recommendations. Most recently, in 2020, CTTI launched its vision for clinical trials in 2030 to provide a path for moving forward. She referred participants to the CTTI website for links to its recommendations, tools, and publications.[10]

Change takes time, and as an example, Tenaerts showed the time line of the ongoing efforts to implement a central IRB process for multi-center clinical trials from 2006 to the present. To help enable change, CTTI launched Building Better Clinical Trials: A Case Study Exchange, a database through which organizations can learn how others have implemented CTTI recommendations and tools.[11] The exchange has case studies from more than 30 organizations that are willing to share how they have used CTTI resources to improve clinical trial efficiency.

Short-Term Goals to Ensure a More Resilient, Sustainable, and Transparent Clinical Trials Enterprise: Panel and Breakout Discussion Highlights

Following the panel discussion, online participants were divided into virtual Zoom breakout rooms to consider short-term, tangible, measurable goals and actions to ensure a more resilient, sustainable, and transparent clinical trials enterprise, and to discuss relevant technologies, tools, techniques, and models that could be used to support this transformation. Upon reconvening in plenary session, Austin and several participants reflected on the panel and breakout group discussions and highlighted the following themes, as described below.

Improving Outreach

Participants discussed ways to improve community outreach and engagement with patients and clinicians. Elena Rios of the National Hispanic Medical Association listed PCORI, the NIH All of Us research program, the Veterans Health Administration, and the teaching clinics of the Health Resources and Services Administration (HRSA) as examples of organizations with connections to communities with diverse populations. She also suggested NIH could reach out to HBCUs and HRSA-designated Hispanic Centers of Excellence to elevate the importance of clinical research in their communities. Partnering with patient advocacy organizations that are already connected to patients was also suggested,

---

[10] See https://www.ctti-clinicaltrials.org (accessed July 1, 2021).
[11] See https://connects.ctti-clinicaltrials.org/case_study_exchange (accessed July 1, 2021).

as well as engaging pharmacists, social workers, and others who have frequent patient contact. The need for a public information campaign about what clinical trials are and the advantages of participation was also reiterated during the discussions. It was also suggested that a patient-friendly source for clinical trial enrollment information is needed.

Shifting the Academic Culture in the United States

Discussion of the U.S. academic culture as it relates to the clinical trials enterprise continued in the breakout groups. As relayed by Austin, participants emphasized the need for change in the academic system for appointments, promotions, and tenure so that participation by academic research faculty in collaborative clinical studies and team-based research is recognized and rewarded. Recalling the discussion of the RECOVERY trial by Landray, Austin pointed out that nearly all practitioners in the United Kingdom are part of the NHS. In the absence of such a centralized system facilitating clinical research in the United States, some individuals proposed creating a separate but affiliated system for clinical research, Austin said, which would not be part of the tenured academic system.

It was suggested that the Association of American Medical Colleges (AAMC) and the National Academies collaborate to consider how the current academic system could better reward the contributions of faculty who recruit participants for clinical trials, especially from underrepresented groups, and how to make clinical research a more appealing career path. Ross McKinney of AAMC agreed that structural change at academic medical centers could help, but added that there are challenges inherent to such change. Other suggestions were that grants could include metrics for community engagement and recruitment to quantify success and recognize achievement, and that recruiting for clinical trials as part of routine care could be part of quality metrics for practices.

Robert Califf pointed out that clinical practices are now commonly part of large health care systems, and many of these systems are now associated with medical schools. He described these large health systems as being partitioned into academic faculty and practitioners that are governed by distinct rules and expectations with little opportunity to work together. The leaders of these systems need to be held accountable for creating a more collaborative environment, he said.

Supporting Providers and Practice-Based Research Networks

There was much discussion of the challenges and barriers to incorporating clinical research into clinical care. Califf cautioned that providers are already overburdened, and adding clinical trials to a practitioner's responsibilities should not further strain the provision of care. A participant added that many providers simply do not have the time to explain a clinical trial opportunity to a patient in the course of a caregiving encounter. Austin agreed and said the academic medical centers in the NCATS Clinical and Translational Science Awards program have links with community centers and practice-based research networks, but these remote sites have limited resources and research capacity. Participants also discussed how busy clinicians might be more effectively engaged in formulating clinical research questions during the early stages of trial development.

Lana Skirboll of Sanofi observed that being an investigator for a clinical trial does not fit into a health care business model in which providers are rewarded based on the volume of patients seen or procedures completed. Hannah Valantine of Stanford University agreed and said that stakeholders in clinical trials (e.g., NIH, PCORI, payers, industry) need to collaborate on shaping "a major systems change," including finding ways to make better use of the existing resources. Barbara Bierer supported remodeling the current system, but noted her concern about creating a separate or parallel system for clinical trials. She observed that many community health centers are not formally linked to an academic health center and said HRSA and CMS should also be included in discussions of the clinical trials enterprise.

Long-Term Goals to Ensure a More Resilient, Sustainable, and Transparent Clinical Trials Enterprise: Panel and Breakout Discussion Highlights

In this breakout session, groups considered longer-term, tangible, measurable goals and actions to ensure a more resilient, sustainable, transparent clinical trials enterprise, and discussed relevant technologies, tools, techniques, and models that could be used to support this transformation. Upon reconvening in plenary session, ElZarrad reflected on the panel and breakout group discussions and highlighted the following themes:

- **Committing resources to a community-based trials system.** There was discussion throughout the workshop about community-based clinical trials and incorporating research seamlessly into routine practice. Participants discussed the role of dedicated resources and funding to build and support the infrastructure for such a system, ElZarrad reported.
- **Engaging payers.** Participants discussed public and private payers as important stakeholders in creating a community-based trials

system. It was pointed out, ElZarrad said, that payers could contribute substantially to discussions of integrating research into care and building efficient systems that generate evidence of value.
- **Eliminating underpowered, uninformative trials.** Participants discussed tools and mechanisms to limit the conduct of clinical trials that are not designed to produce robust data. The role of journals as partners in ensuring the quality of published trials was mentioned, ElZarrad said, and it was pointed out that there has been a proliferation of journals that perpetuate the dissemination of bad information from poorly conducted trials. Valda Vinson of *Science* suggested that more information clearly articulating characteristics of high-quality pragmatic trials could be helpful for journals and peer reviewers.
- **Informing the media and the public about clinical trials and trial quality.** Participants discussed the importance of publicizing positive examples of well-designed, well-executed clinical trials, ElZarrad said, and working with the media to improve the quality of reporting on clinical trials.

REFLECTIONS ON RESILIENCE, SUSTAINABILITY, AND TRANSPARENCY OF THE CLINICAL TRIALS ENTERPRISE

To close this part of the workshop, Krofah and Steven Galson reflected on the key messages they heard during the discussions.

- Pragmatic, randomized controlled trials can achieve diverse and inclusive enrollment, as demonstrated by the RECOVERY trial, but there is still much progress to be made, Krofah said. Who is recruited is directly impacted by where clinical trial sites are located, and this could be addressed by designing more community-based trials. The roles of technology and decentralized trials in expanding inclusivity were also discussed.
- For community-based trials to be sustainable, participating as investigators must be worthwhile for community health care providers, and appropriate incentives can drive more participation, Krofah said.
- Trust and transparency are core elements of a transformed 2030 clinical trials enterprise, Krofah summarized. Participants discussed leveraging existing relationships and building on shared values to establish trust of the clinical trials enterprise within the community. Galson added that the tools for creating more transparency exist, and highlighted workshop participants' calls for prioritizing it.

- Patients are the experts in their disease, but participants asked: Is the clinical trials enterprise listening to patients? There was much discussion about improving outreach and engaging patients in the trial process from the start of study development to understand what matters to them. "Invest in building longitudinal relationships and come to the community well before you need those participants to enroll in the trial," Krofah said, recalling the panel discussions.
- There are impediments and disincentives to progress that are inherent in the clinical trials system, Galson reported (e.g., the current academic culture in the United States). However, discussions trended toward transforming the current trials system rather than creating an entirely separate system for clinical trials.
- A coordinated, central plan for transforming the clinical trials enterprise could be a beneficial next step, Krofah concluded, drawing from the discussion by Lewis-Hall. A multi-stakeholder approach to developing such a plan could ensure that all voices are represented in the effort to create a more inclusive clinical trials enterprise. "We cannot do this in our own individual siloes," she said. Galson highlighted the importance of including experts in social sciences in these discussions as well. Participants discussed a role for the National Academies in convening stakeholders from across the clinical trials ecosystem to develop a national action plan.

6

Opportunities for Transformation

> **Highlights of Key Points Made by Individual Speakers**
> - Elements of success toward more inclusive clinical trials involve building community trust in the research enterprise, encouraging the patient perspective in the early stages of trial development, and making it easier for people to participate. (McClellan)
> - There are opportunities to facilitate change in the clinical trials enterprise by building upon ongoing public health policy activities (e.g., Prescription Drug User Fee Act [PDUFA] program reauthorization). (McClellan)
> - "New innovations need to be … pressure tested to ensure that the innovation works within our clinical trials ecosystem in a way that continues to ensure patient safety and integrity of the underlying dataset." (Abernethy)
> - The technology industry should be included in stakeholder discussions as a partner in envisioning how the clinical trials enterprise can evolve for the future in terms of technical and data capabilities, not just as vendors providing services. (Abernethy)
> - In a public health emergency, the goal of the clinical trials enterprise should be to rapidly generate robust, actionable data that can be used to improve standards of care and disease outcomes. However, the response of the U.S. clinical

trials ecosystem to the pandemic was less than optimal. (Woodcock)
- The creation of a community-based clinical trials network is as essential to pandemic preparedness as ensuring the availability of personal protective equipment, and therefore, should be a government-supported activity. "We need a national clinical trial capacity stockpile, just as we need a stockpile of medicine and equipment." (Woodcock)
- Many lessons can be learned from what worked and what did not in the clinical trials response to the COVID-19 pandemic. (Abernethy, McClellan, Woodcock)

Over the course of the workshop, current and former FDA officials shared their personal perspectives on the current state of the clinical trials enterprise; the unique opportunity to learn from how product development unfolded during the COVID-19 pandemic response; and how to realize the vision of a more efficient, effective, person-centered, and inclusive clinical trials enterprise that is integrated with routine health care delivery.[1]

OPPORTUNITIES TO TRANSFORM THE CLINICAL TRIALS ENTERPRISE

Mark McClellan, director of the Duke–Margolis Center for Health Policy and former FDA commissioner and former CMS administrator, shared his perspective on opportunities to transform the clinical trials enterprise in a conversation moderated by Amy Abernethy.

Creating More Person-Centered and Accessible Clinical Trials

"There is … broad awareness that we ought to be able to do better," McClellan said, referring to creating a more person-centered and easily accessible clinical trials enterprise. He referenced the CTTI vision for the clinical trials ecosystem and beyond: transforming clinical trials for 2030,[2] which outlines directions for the future (also discussed in Chapter 5).

One approach to increasing patient-centeredness in clinical trials is to integrate trials into routine health care, McClellan said. Integrating data

---

[1] McClellan and Abernethy spoke at the meeting on May 11, 2021. Janet Woodcock, acting commissioner of food and drugs, FDA, spoke at the meeting on January 26, 2021.

[2] For more information, see https://www.ctti-clinicaltrials.org/transforming-trials-2030 (accessed August 3, 2021).

collection and care delivery processes would also align with another key interest of health care organizations: lowering costs. Reimbursement is shifting toward patient-centered, results-based payments (e.g., improving diabetes outcomes) and away from traditional fee-for-service payments, he said. To make this transition, health systems are, for example, investing in medical record integration, developing new team-based approaches to care, and using digital health technologies to remotely monitor patients and support self-management of disease.

The transformation of the clinical trials enterprise continues to move forward during the ongoing response to a pandemic, and McClellan and Abernethy discussed "using the pandemic as a proof point," learning from what worked and what did not when it comes to simplifying trial designs and integrating clinical research and practice. McClellan pointed to presentations by Martin Landray and others, who described the design and implementation of trials during the pandemic, which enrolled diverse participant populations (e.g., the RECOVERY trial). As another example, he mentioned the NIH Accelerating COVID-19 Therapeutic Interventions and Vaccines (ACTIV) public–private partnership[3] to test new therapeutics and vaccines for effectiveness in treating COVID-19. He described the ACTIV-6 trial[4] as "fully distributed" and intentionally designed to be integrated into community-based care. There are positive lessons from those examples on how to efficiently identify and engage potential trial participants, improve the informed consent process, and design trials that are fit-for-purpose and not unnecessarily burdensome for clinicians. Sufficient data will need to be collected to define the safety profile of interventions and characterize patient responses, he said, whether the interventions are new molecular entities or repurposed drug products. Abernethy summarized that clinical trials conducted within the context of clinical care should still provide robust answers to key questions and keep patients safe, all while increasing efficiency overall.

Building Trust and Engaging Communities

Building community trust in the research enterprise and including the patient perspective in the early stages of trial development are "hallmarks" of clinical trials that have been successfully inclusive of diverse populations, McClellan said. He noted that this concept is discussed in the

---

[3] For more information, see https://www.nih.gov/research-training/medical-research-initiatives/activ (accessed August 1, 2021).

[4] For more information, see https://www.nih.gov/research-training/medical-research-initiatives/activ/covid-19-therapeutics-prioritized-testing-clinical-trials#activ6 (accessed August 3, 2021).

CTTI vision statement for 2030[5] as part of building more patient-centered and easily accessible trials.

McClellan observed that some of the early COVID-19 trials recruited participants through existing academic clinical networks and, as a result, did not successfully enroll participants. Abernethy emphasized that trials should "meet people where they are" by making it easier for health systems and the organizations that serve them to participate at trial sites. McClellan discussed two approaches for better engaging patients in the community.

- **Simplify existing trial networks.** Consider how trial networks could be adapted to reach broader populations using the tools and technologies discussed at the workshop to improve regulatory interactions, IRB oversight, and frontline clinician training. Abernethy described this as "wicking away the work" to reduce the burden for community health care providers who must balance enrolling a patient in a clinical trial against other tasks and payment incentives.
- **Leverage capacity outside of the clinical trials enterprise.** Capacities for longitudinal patient tracking are already being deployed on the care delivery side. There are "increasingly sophisticated electronic registries powered by payment reforms and performance accountability around improving outcomes," McClellan explained. Federally qualified health centers, accountable care organizations, and other health organizations that serve more vulnerable communities are using longitudinal patient tracking for quality improvement and for targeting interventions (e.g., identifying patients who might benefit from telehealth services). Additionally, there is a growing base of reliable longitudinal information on characteristics of patients with common chronic diseases, which may include data on characteristics that may not be captured through clinical trials (e.g., housing status, food insecurity), but are relevant for health outcomes.

Facilitating Action Through Government Support and Coordination

A key role for government is to be a facilitator of the actions discussed throughout the workshop, McClellan said. He added that there are opportunities to facilitate change in the clinical trials enterprise by building on ongoing public health policy activities. For example, the

---

[5] For more information, see https://ctti-clinicaltrials.org/who_we_are/transforming-trials-2030 (accessed April 13, 2022).

reauthorization of PDUFA provides an opportunity for FDA to promote more comprehensive and coordinated data collection. Another opportunity is, as discussed, learning from what did and did not work during the COVID-19 pandemic response, especially around rapidly mobilizing for evidence generation. Federal agencies other than FDA taking action in this area could also include NIH and the Biomedical Advanced Research and Development Authority.

As drug discovery, development, and translation have evolved, pre- and postmarket evidence generation has become more of a continuum, McClellan pointed out. This is related, in part, to FDA's accelerated product approval pathways for breakthrough treatments that address serious unmet medical needs. But it is also about putting into practice the concept of a learning health care system. He noted that the federal government is interested in policy changes that support the collection of better postmarket data and the translation of that data into health care practice. For example, CMS called for public comment on a new Medicare coverage pathway, Medicare Coverage of Innovative Technology,[6] for FDA-designated breakthrough medical devices, and he anticipated this may inform development of new policies related to federal support for registries or other platforms for collecting evidence after marketing approval. McClellan also highlighted the opportunity to update policies that cover advanced diagnostics, including artificial intelligence– and big data–informed diagnostic capabilities. This area could benefit from the ability to leverage real-world evidence and, potentially, to randomize populations for evidence collection in the postmarket setting.

In closing, McClellan emphasized that it is easier for the federal government to act on an issue when there is strong stakeholder support for taking action. Cross-stakeholder consensus and support are needed not only from FDA and research-funding agencies, but also from agencies that engage in and benefit from evidence generation in the postmarket space, such as CMS and The Office of the National Coordinator for Health Information Technology. Abernethy agreed and summarized that "there is a confluence of activity" occurring across federal agencies, but there is a need for support from across the clinical trials stakeholder community.

INNOVATING FOR 2030 NOW

Abernethy offered seven key points to keep in mind as the clinical trials enterprise innovates toward the future. The year "2030 is now," she

---

[6] For more information, see https://www.cms.gov/newsroom/fact-sheets/medicare-coverage-innovative-technology-cms-3372-f (accessed August 4, 2021).

said, stressing that the vision for 2030 is unfolding in 2021 and stems from the actions and innovations of today and the coming years.

1. **Ensuring all stakeholders are at the table.** This includes clinical trialists, manufacturers, patients, end users (e.g., quantitative scientists, biostatisticians), technologists, and others. Importantly, Abernethy said, stakeholders need to learn how to talk to each other, as well as how to listen. "How do we make sure that we have all actors at the table, and that we have an equal power dynamic with equal voice?" she asked.
2. **Including technology experts as partners.** Abernethy emphasized that the technology industry should be included in stakeholder discussions as partners, rather than simply as vendors providing services. Technology partners can help envision how the clinical trials enterprise can evolve for the future in terms of technical and data capabilities, she said.
3. **Ensuring patient-centricity.** Clinical trials test new interventions and involve risk for participants. It is important to incorporate patient input and keep patient safety at the forefront of clinical trials, "not in a paternalistic way, but in a way that is a conversation," Abernethy said. She added that maintaining a focus on participant safety also helps promote trust.
4. **Remembering the goal of research is generating data.** She observed that sometimes there is more attention on the specific technology being used (e.g., telehealth capabilities) rather than the quality of the data being generated. "We need to make sure that the datasets that get generated have the kind of integrity and quality and consistency of data that we are going to need to make confident decisions … about the medical product or health care intervention that is being studied," Abernethy said. The focus should be on how best to obtain, validate, and use the clinical data that are relevant for the intervention being investigated. For example, trial sponsors, researchers, and regulators could consider whether traceability to source data is needed in specific circumstances, or whether EHR or claims data can be merged with data generated within a clinical trial to build the needed dataset.
5. **Looking for new and innovative ways to solve problems and develop capabilities for the future.** As examples, Abernethy mentioned innovations such as tokenization of health data, privacy-sparing innovations, and synthetic datasets. She added that "new innovations need to be … pressure tested to ensure that the innovation works within our clinical trials ecosystem in a way that continues to ensure patient safety and integrity of the underlying dataset."

6. **Ensuring that stakeholders in the clinical trials ecosystem are aware of and understand the new capabilities being deployed.** Abernethy emphasized that regulatory agencies, in particular, need to have the opportunity to familiarize themselves with new capabilities being used in clinical trials and to ensure they work as expected and intended within the clinical trials infrastructure. She emphasized that this process of building familiarity builds trust in the new capabilities and infrastructure.
7. **Focusing on the ultimate goal of informing better health care decisions.** The clinical trials infrastructure exists to generate the clinical evidence needed to make decisions about health-related interventions. To be relevant and useful for this task, the clinical trials infrastructure must function as expected; be inclusive to the extent possible; engage stakeholders, including trial participants, in the process; maximize trial participant safety while advancing cutting-edge medical product development; and generate credible, high-quality datasets that can inform decisions and assessments of the medical intervention being studied, Abernethy summarized.

TAKING THE LESSONS FROM THE COVID-19 PANDEMIC RESPONSE FORWARD

Janet Woodcock, acting commissioner of food and drugs, FDA shared her perspective on the current status of the clinical trials ecosystem, discussing the response to the COVID-19 pandemic as a case example, and suggested key actions for moving forward.

Studying the COVID-19 Pandemic Response as a Model

In a public health emergency, such as the COVID-19 pandemic, the goal of the clinical trials enterprise should be to rapidly generate robust, actionable data that can be used to improve standards of care and disease outcomes, Woodcock said. However, the response of the U.S. clinical trials ecosystem to the pandemic was less than optimal. Woodcock reported that more than 500 small therapeutic trials were initiated in the United States, many of which were non-randomized. Only about 5 percent of the trial arms were adequately powered to yield actionable data (i.e., data that are useful to regulators or clinical guideline developers). Many trials were redundant (i.e., numerous small studies testing the same compounds), and many did not achieve rapid or complete enrollment (Bugin and Woodcock, 2021). "In a crisis, we are left with a lot less evidence than we could have had, and that the system could have delivered, had it been more organized, more focused on the societal goal, and generally more effective," Woodcock said.

Woodcock suggested that the clinical trials response to the pandemic be studied as a model of the larger clinical trials system in general, which also suffers from barriers to evidence development and clinical evaluation. She noted that discussions of these problems have been ongoing for more than a decade. Still, many remain comfortable with the status quo and there has been little motivation for change. She described the failure to rapidly generate actionable data during the COVID-19 pandemic as "the expected outcome of the system that we have." What is needed now is an understanding of what contributed to this outcome, followed by efforts to make substantive changes. For example, there are lessons to be learned about site selection from the use of academic medical centers for COVID-19 clinical trials. Woodcock said that conducting clinical research primarily at academic medical centers results in competition for patients, study staff, and other resources, which can slow study progress and limit evidence generation. At the same time, many of those who have the disease being studied receive their health care in other settings and are not afforded the opportunity to participate in, and possibly benefit from, a clinical study.

Building a Community-Based Trials Network

To enable the clinical trials enterprise to be better prepared for the next public health emergency, Woodcock proposed building a community-based clinical trials network. Having such a network in place before there is urgent need will allow for increased community participation in clinical research during a public health emergency. Community-based clinical trial sites could be supported by specialized CROs, for example, and procedural and monitoring costs could be reduced by engaging a central IRB and collecting data from EHRs.

Woodcock said the creation of a community-based clinical trials network is as essential to pandemic preparedness as ensuring the availability of personal protective equipment, and thus should be a government-supported activity. "We need a national clinical trial capacity stockpile, just as we need a stockpile of medicine and equipment," she said. She emphasized the need to regularly use such a network between emergencies to ensure it has the functional capacity needed to efficiently and effectively generate evidence. This could be done by, for example, conducting studies that answer pressing societal health questions and generate actionable evidence (e.g., studies to improve the treatment of chronic and neglected diseases). The questions, she concluded, are "Will we be prepared next time? Will we be able to respond and learn very quickly the best treatments for our patients if this happens again?"

CLOSING REMARKS

At the end of the final part of the workshop, Esther Krofah and Steven Galson reflected on the discussions that took place over the course of the workshop, which unexpectedly spanned 5 months due to the COVID-19 pandemic and the need to hold the workshop virtually. Krofah believed there was a strong sense that the experience of the COVID-19 public health crisis had created momentum for change. The discussions at the workshop were informed and influenced by the collective pandemic experience of the workshop participants, and many actionable steps toward achieving a transformed clinical trials enterprise for 2030 were discussed. Krofah noted that the U.S. government is undertaking efforts to learn from the experiences of COVID-19 clinical trials, and there are lessons to be learned and leads to follow from the CTTI vision for clinical trials in 2030 and the efforts of the TransCelerate biopharmaceutical member companies. Galson said a silver lining in the pandemic response is the ability to learn from "the real-life examples of the problems with our chronic lack of inclusiveness, and our challenges with bringing people together in a way that creates data that are actually useful for the health care system." He urged participants to take advantage of the momentum and apply these lessons now to transform the clinical trials enterprise for the coming decade.

References

AstraZeneca. 2020. *Clinical study protocol—amendment 2 AZD1222-D8110C00001.* https://s3.amazonaws.com/ctr-med-7111/D8110C00001/52bec400-80f6-4c1b-8791-0483923d0867/c8070a4e-6a9d-46f9-8c32-cece903592b9/D8110C00001_CSP-v2.pdf (accessed August 3, 2021).

Baxter, R., N. Taylor, I. Kellar, and R. Lawton. 2016. What methods are used to apply positive deviance within healthcare organisations? A systematic review. *BMJ Quality & Safety* 25(3):190–201.

Bugin, K., and J. Woodcock. 2021. Trends in COVID-19 therapeutic clinical trials. *Nature Review Drug Discovery* 20:254–255.

CDC (Centers for Disease Control and Prevention). 2021. *Risk for COVID-19 infection, hospitalization, and death by race/ethnicity.* https://www.cdc.gov/coronavirus/2019-ncov/covid-data/investigations-discovery/hospitalization-death-by-race-ethnicity.html (accessed August 3, 2021).

Collins, R., L. Bowman, M. Landray, and R. Peto. 2020. The magic of randomization versus the myth of real-world evidence. *New England Journal of Medicine* 382(7):674–678.

COVID R&D Alliance. 2021. https://www.covidrdalliance.com (accessed August 3, 2021).

Emanuel, E. J., C. Zhang, and A. Diana. 2020. Where is America's groundbreaking COVID-19 research? The U.S. could learn a lot from Britain. *The New York Times*, September 1, https://www.nytimes.com/2020/09/01/opinion/coronavirus-clinical-research.html (accessed July 1, 2021).

FDA (U.S. Food and Drug Administration). 2020a. *Conduct of clinical trials of medical products during the COVID-19 public health emergency: Guidance for industry, investigators, and institutional review boards.* https://www.fda.gov/media/136238/download (accessed August 3, 2021).

FDA. 2020b. *Drug trials snapshots summary report 2015–2019.* https://www.fda.gov/media/143592/download (accessed August 3, 2021).

IOM (Institute of Medicine). 2012. *Envisioning a transformed clinical trials enterprise in the United States: Establishing an agenda for 2020: Workshop summary.* Washington, DC: The National Academies Press.

Janssen Vaccines and Prevention. 2020. *VAC31518 (JNJ-78436735) clinical protocol VAC31518COV3001 amendment 1.* https://www.jnj.com/coronavirus/covid-19-phase-3-study-clinical-protocol (accessed August 3, 2021).

Korn, E., B. Freidlin, M. Mooney, and J. S. Abrams. 2010. Accrual experience of National Cancer Institute Cooperative Group phase III trials activated from 2000 to 2007. *Journal of Clinical Oncology* 28(35):5197–5201.

Moderna TX. 2020. *Protocol mRNA-1273-P301, amendment 3.* https://www.modernatx.com/sites/default/files/mRNA-1273-P301-Protocol.pdf (accessed August 3, 2021).

NASEM (National Academies of Sciences, Engineering, and Medicine). 2018. *Advancing the science of patient input in medical product R&D: Towards a research agenda: Proceedings of a workshop—in brief.* Washington, DC: The National Academies Press.

NASEM. 2020. *The role of digital health technologies in drug development: Proceedings of a workshop.* Washington, DC: The National Academies Press.

NCHS (National Center for Health Statistics). 2021. *Health, United States, 2019: Tables 14, 22, 26.* https://www.cdc.gov/nchs/hus/contents2019.htm (accessed August 3, 2021).

Pfizer Inc. 2020. *PF-07302048 (BNT162 RNA-based COVID-19 vaccines) protocol C4591001.* https://cdn.pfizer.com/pfizercom/2020-11/C4591001_Clinical_Protocol_Nov2020.pdf (accessed August 3, 2021).

Steinhubl, S. R., D. L. Wolff-Hughes, W. Nilsen, E. Iturriaga, and R. M. Califf. 2019. Digital clinical trials: Creating a vision for the future. *npj Digital Medicine* 2:126.

TransCelerate (TransCelerate Biopharma Inc.). 2020. *COVID-19 data sharing via DataCelerate.* https://www.transceleratebiopharmainc.com/covid-19 (accessed August 3, 2021).

Appendix A

Health Affairs Blog Posts

The blog posts associated with the Envisioning a Transformed Clinical Trials Enterprise for 2030 virtual workshop (listed below) are available at https://www.healthaffairs.org/topic/ss170 (accessed July 1, 2021).[1]

- *Transforming Clinical Trials: A New Vision for 2030.* In this blog post, Marilyn Metcalf and Rob Weker lay out their vision for person-centered clinical trials in the year 2030 and provide an outline of how to get there.
- *Driving Towards More Inclusive Clinical Trials by 2030: Action Without Strategy Is Aimless, Strategy Without Action Is Powerless.* Silas Buchanan lays out a vision for a clinical trials enterprise that benefits from diversity in its participants and workforce through ongoing community engagement.
- *The Future of Clinical Trials: How Will New Technologies Affect the Lives of Participants?* Andy Coravos, Eric Perakslis, and Sam Roosz envision how the lives of four fictional individuals could be changed with the integration of technologies into the clinical trials enterprise.
- *A Future of Trusted Clinical Trials: Communication Strategies to Encourage Trust and Transparency.* Brian Southwell discusses the

---

[1] These *Health Affairs* blog posts represent the opinions of the authors and do not necessarily represent the views of any one organization; the Forum on Drug Discovery, Development, and Translation; or the National Academies, and were not subjected to the review procedures of, nor are a publication or product of, the National Academies.

importance of fostering trust and transparency in the clinical trials enterprise for improving the person-centeredness and relevance of clinical trial research.
- *Clinical Trials in Crisis: Building on COVID-19's Lessons Toward a Better Future.* Esther Krofah, Steven Galson, Robert Califf, and Gregory Simon synthesize three central categories emerging from these workshop discussions for future improvement—engagement, efficiency, and coordination—and issue a call to action.

Appendix B

Speaker and Moderator Biographies

Amy Abernethy, M.D., Ph.D., is an oncologist and an internationally recognized clinical data expert and clinical researcher. As the former principal deputy commissioner of food and drugs, Dr. Abernethy helped oversee the U.S. Food and Drug Administration's (FDA's) day-to-day functioning and directs special and high-priority, cross-cutting initiatives that impact the regulation of drugs, medical devices, tobacco, and food. As former acting chief information officer, she oversaw FDA's data and technical vision as well as its execution. She has held multiple executive roles at Flatiron Health and was a professor of medicine at the Duke University School of Medicine, where she ran the Center for Learning Health Care and the Duke Cancer Care Research Program. Dr. Abernethy received her M.D. at Duke University, where she did her internal medicine residency, served as the chief resident, and completed her hematology/oncology fellowship. She received her Ph.D. from Flinders University and her B.A. from the University of Pennsylvania and is boarded in palliative medicine.

Anita LaFrance Allen, J.D., Ph.D., is an internationally renowned expert on privacy law and ethics and is recognized for her contributions to legal philosophy, women's rights, and diversity in higher education. In 2013, Dr. Allen was appointed the University of Pennsylvania's vice provost for faculty, and, in 2015, the chair of the Penn Provost's Advisory Council on Arts, Culture and the Humanities. From 2010 to 2017, she served on President Obama's Presidential Commission for the Study of Bioethical

Issues. She was presented the Lifetime Achievement Award of the Electronic Privacy Information Center in 2015 and elected to the National Academy of Medicine in 2016.

In 2017, Dr. Allen was elected the vice president/president-elect of the Eastern Division of the American Philosophical Association. In 2015, Dr. Allen was on the summer faculty of the School of Criticism and Theory at Cornell University. A 2-year term as an associate of the Johns Hopkins Humanities Center concluded in 2018. Her books include *Unpopular Privacy: What Must We Hide* (Oxford, 2011); *Privacy Law and Society* (Thomson/West, 2017); *The New Ethics: A Guided Tour of the 21st Century Moral Landscape* (Miramax/Hyperion, 2004); and *Why Privacy Isn't Everything: Feminist Reflections on Personal Accountability* (Rowman & Littlefield, 2003).

Margaret Anderson, M.S., is a managing director at Deloitte Consulting, serving clients at the intersection of the nonprofit sector, federal health agencies, and the life sciences industry. She is also the leader of diversity, equity, and inclusion for Deloitte's Strategy & Analytics. Her career as a strategist has traversed roles in a variety of settings, always putting patients at the center. She joined Deloitte from FasterCures, where she helped set up the organization and served as the executive director. She began at the Congressional Office of Technology Assessment, studying the impact of the mapping of the human genome on our lives. She currently sits on a number of boards, including Act for the National Institutes of Health, Allen Institute, FasterCures, Friends of Cancer Research, and the Melanoma Research Alliance.

RADM Richardae Araojo, Pharm.D., M.S., serves as the associate commissioner for minority health and the director of the Office of Minority Health and Health Equity at the U.S. Food and Drug Administration (FDA). In this role, RADM Araojo provides leadership, oversight, and direction on minority health and health disparity matters for FDA. RADM Araojo previously served as the director of the Office of Medical Policy Initiatives in FDA's Center for Drug Evaluation and Research (CDER), where she led a variety of broad-based medical and clinical policy initiatives to improve the science and efficiency of clinical trials and enhance professional and patient labeling. RADM Araojo joined FDA in 2003, where she held several positions in CDER. RADM Araojo received her Pharm.D. from Virginia Commonwealth University, completed a pharmacy practice residency at the University of Maryland, and earned an M.S. in pharmacy regulation and policy from the University of Florida.

Christopher P. Austin, M.D., joined Flagship Pioneering in 2021 as a chief executive officer (CEO) partner. Dr. Austin is part of the broader Flagship senior leadership team, participating in Flagship leadership meetings, serving on selected Flagship company boards, and providing his experience across the ecosystem. Dr. Austin will also serve as the CEO of a Flagship-founded company currently in stealth, to be announced at a later date. He is a trained clinician and geneticist, with more than 20 years of experience in translational research in the public and private sectors. He joins Flagship from the National Institutes of Health (NIH), where he served as the founding director of the National Center for Advancing Translational Sciences (NCATS). In this role, he led NCATS's work to transform translation—the process by which interventions that benefit patients are developed and deployed—from an empirical process into a predictive science. Dr. Austin previously served as the senior advisor to the director for translational research at NIH's National Human Genome Research Institute, implementing research programs to derive scientific insights and therapeutic benefits from the results of the Human Genome Project. He also founded and directed NIH's Chemical Genomics Center, Therapeutics for Rare and Neglected Diseases program, Toxicology in the 21st Century initiative, and Center for Translational Therapeutics. Before joining NIH, Dr. Austin worked at Merck, where he directed programs on genome-based discovery of novel targets and drugs, with a particular focus on treatments for schizophrenia and Alzheimer's disease. He is a member of the National Academy of Medicine and earned his M.D. from Harvard Medical School and his A.B. in biology from Princeton University. He completed a research fellowship in developmental neurogenetics at Harvard University and trained in internal medicine and neurology at the Massachusetts General Hospital.

Jan Benedikt Brönneke, LL.M., is the director of law and economics of health technologies of the German health innovation hub (hih)—the Federal Health Ministry's think tank on the digitalization of health care. As a trained lawyer and economist with a research background in medical law, health technology assessment, and medical device regulation, he is leading, among others, hih's projects on matters of access, regulation, evaluation, and reimbursement of digital technologies within the German statutory health insurance system. In this position he was closely supporting the development and implementation of the German Digital Healthcare Act, the Patient Data Protection Act, and other legislative activities regarding digitalization of the German health care system. Before joining hih, he worked for the Federal Joint Committee on quality assurance in hospitals and private practices and was a manager for a Berlin-based law firm specializing in the law of medical devices and pharmaceuticals. With this background, he bridges the gaps among disciplines as well as regulatory authorities and private actors, such as technology developers, doctors, and hospitals.

Dyan Bryson, M.B.A., is a life science industry sales and marketing veteran who has consistently developed innovative initiatives that have helped to propel the industry forward. In the past decade, Ms. Bryson's mantra has been that patients should be part of the drug development process from before the Investigational New Drug stage through commercialization, years ahead of the U.S. Food and Drug Administration's Patient-Focused Drug Development effort.

Examples of the initiatives Ms. Bryson has led include

- For Merck–Medco, developed one of the industry's first patient services hubs.
- For Merck, led the Vioxx launch outside the United States; developed all branding, messaging, and promotional materials.
- For Pfizer Inc. and the American Pain Association, developed the industry's first digital Congress delivery, including Continuing Medical Education accreditation.
- For Sanofi, developed the Community Health Partnership, the industry's first enterprisewide, patient-focused initiative that resulted in a positive change in behavior for both patients and physicians. This initiative was focused on supporting diverse patient populations; all materials were translated and acculturated. On a $3.4 million investment, Ms. Bryson and her team returned $406 million to the brands.
- For Retrophin, ensured patient insights were part of business decisions across the entire company. This resulted in improved diverse clinical trial recruitment, driving a formulation change to ensure wider drug usage among an appropriate rare disease population. Developed a patient advisory board to ensure ongoing patient input to business decisions.
- Ms. Bryson has worked with technology to collect patient-reported outcomes/real-world data to help people manage their health better, help companies go "beyond the brand," and enhance diversity in clinical trials.

Ms. Bryson has won numerous industry awards for her efforts, including being honored as part of the PharmaVoice 100 as a life sciences industry innovator.

Silas Buchanan, B.A., is a passionate and experienced underserved community outreach and engagement strategist. He is dedicated to building partnerships and crafting Web-based ecosystems that solve for known failure points. Mr. Buchanan has worked with various health care payer, provider, government, and academic stakeholders across the United

States and has expertise in recruiting, activating, and connecting with trusted faith- and community-based organizations.

Mr. Buchanan works closely with public and private stakeholders to identify actionable ehealth and mhealth engagement opportunities that also support sustainable broadband adoption and digital inclusion efforts for underserved populations. He has testified before the U.S. Department of Health and Human Services' Health Information Technology Policy Committee, Meaningful Use Workgroup. He was selected as a member of the White House Summit to Achieve eHealth Equity, selected as the co-chair of the Awareness Committee for Region V of the National Partnership for Action to End Health Disparities, and recently selected as an inaugural National Advisory Board member of the Morehouse School of Medicine's National COVID-19 Resiliency Network. In addition, he is an inaugural member of the National eHealth Collaborative Consumer Committee and a member of the Ohio Patient-Centered Primary Care Collaborative.

Howard A. Burris III, M.D., serves as the president and the chief medical officer of Sarah Cannon, as well as the executive director of drug development for the research institute. He is an associate of Tennessee Oncology, PLLC, where he practices medical oncology. Dr. Burris's clinical research career has focused on the development of new cancer agents, with an emphasis on first-in-human therapies, having led the trials of many novel antibodies, small molecules, and chemotherapies that are now approved by the U.S. Food and Drug Administration, including ado-trastuzumab emtansine, everolimus, and gemcitabine. In 1997, he established in Nashville the first community-based, early-phase drug development program, which grew into the Sarah Cannon Research Institute. He has authored more than 400 publications and 700 abstracts. Sarah Cannon has now dosed more than 350 first-in-human anticancer therapies and enrolls more than 3,000 patients per year into clinical trials. Dr. Burris served as the elected president of the American Society of Clinical Oncology (ASCO) in 2019–2020. He also currently serves on the Board of ASCO's Conquer Cancer Foundation. Additionally in 2014, Dr. Burris was selected by his peers as a Giant of Cancer Care for his achievements in drug development.

Dr. Burris completed his undergraduate education at the U.S. Military Academy at West Point, his M.D. at the University of South Alabama, and his internal medicine residency and oncology fellowship at Brooke Army Medical Center in San Antonio. While in Texas, he also served as the director of clinical research at the Institute for Drug Development of the Cancer Therapy and Research Center and The University of Texas Health Science Center. He attained the rank of lieutenant colonel in the U.S. Army, and among his decorations he was awarded a Meritorious Service Medal with oak leaf cluster for his service in Operation Joint Endeavor.

Robert Califf, M.D., MACC, is the head of clinical policy and strategy for Verily Life Sciences and Google Health for Verily and Google Health. Prior to this Dr. Califf was the vice chancellor for health data science for the Duke University School of Medicine; the director of Duke Forge, Duke's center for health data science; and the Donald F. Fortin, M.D. Professor of Cardiology. He served as the deputy commissioner for medical products and tobacco in the U.S. Food and Drug Administration (FDA) from 2015 to 2016, and as the commissioner from 2016 to 2017. A nationally and internationally recognized leader in cardiovascular medicine, health outcomes research, health care quality, and clinical research, Dr. Califf is a graduate of the Duke University School of Medicine. Dr. Califf was the founding director of the Duke Clinical Research Institute and is one of the most frequently cited authors in biomedical science.

Janice Chang, M.B.A., is the chief operating officer at TransCelerate BioPharma Inc. She has been involved with the organization since its inception. In her current position, Ms. Chang works closely with the chief executive officer and the Board of Directors to shape the long-term strategic vision and priorities for the organization and its more than 30 initiatives. She defines and guides TransCelerate's overall external engagement strategy with global health authorities, governmental agencies, industry groups, and TransCelerate's country network spanning across 30 countries. She has accountability for overseeing TransCelerate's corporate operations and works closely with her team to drive strategic delivery of TransCelerate's portfolio.

Chang also actively participates in various cross-stakeholder global discussions to help evolve its research and development paradigm. Most recently she joined the Advisory Council for HL7 International's Vulcan Accelerator. Vulcan is a global strategic effort to bring together stakeholders across the translational and clinical research community to align on data exchange standards to bridge existing gaps between clinical care and clinical research, enabling more effective acquisition, exchange, and use of health care data in translational and clinical research.

With a background of more than 20 years of experience leading initiatives in large pharma and biotech companies, Ms. Chang has experience spanning across regulatory, clinical, and manufacturing. She is passionate about driving meaningful change across our ecosystem and not settling for the status quo. She believes in reimagining the way we advance innovative medicine and advocates for the power of open collaboration across stakeholder groups.

Luther T. Clark, M.D., is the deputy chief patient officer and the global director of scientific medical and patient perspective in the Office of the Chief Patient Officer at Merck. In this role, he is responsible for (1) gathering internal and external scientific and medical information to assist with decision making at the highest levels; (2) collaborating across Merck to increase the voice of patients, directly and indirectly, in decision making; (3) collaborating with key internal and external stakeholders in the development of a systematized approach for collecting and incorporating patient insights across the patient journey and product life cycle; and (4) representing Merck externally, expanding bidirectional exchange with key patient and professional leaders and organizations.

Dr. Clark leads Merck's Patient Insights Team, is the co-leader of the team that champions Health Care Equities (including the promotion of health literacy and research diversity), and chairs the Patient Engagement, Health Literacy & Clinical Trials Diversity Investigator Initiated Studies Research Committee.

Prior to joining Merck, Dr. Clark was the chief of the Division of Cardiovascular Medicine at the State University of New York Downstate Medical Center (SUNY Downstate) and the founding director of the National Institutes of Health–funded Brooklyn Health Disparities Research Center. Dr. Clark earned his B.A. from Harvard College and his M.D. from Harvard Medical School. He is a fellow of the American College of Cardiology and the American College of Physicians, and a past member of the Board of Directors of the Founders Affiliate of the American Heart Association. He is a nationally and internationally recognized leader in cardiovascular education, clinical investigation, cardiovascular disease prevention, and health equity. He has authored more than 100 publications and edited and was principal contributor to the textbook *Cardiovascular Disease and Diabetes* (McGraw-Hill).

Dr. Clark has received numerous awards and honors, including the Harvard University Alumni Lifetime Achievement Award for Excellence in Medicine. He is the current president of the Health Science Center at Brooklyn Foundation, SUNY Downstate Medical Center.

Andy Coravos, M.B.A., is the co-founder and the chief executive officer of HumanFirst (previously known as Elektra Labs), building a digital medicine platform with a focus on digital biomarkers for decentralized clinical trials. She is a member of the Harvard–Massachusetts Institute of Technology's Center for Regulatory Sciences. Formerly, Coravos served as an entrepreneur in residence in the digital health unit at the U.S. Food and Drug Administration, focusing on the pre-certification program and policies around software and artificial intelligence/machine learning. Previously, she worked as a software engineer at Akili Interactive Labs, a leading digital therapeutic company. Ms. Coravos also worked at KKR, a private equity firm, and McKinsey & Company, a management consulting firm, where she focused on the health care industry. She serves on the Board of the Digital Medicine Society, and she is an advisor to the Biohacking Village at DEF CON.

M. Khair ElZarrad, Ph.D., M.P.H., is the deputy director of the Office of Medical Policy at the U.S. Food and Drug Administration's (FDA's) Center for Drug Evaluation and Research, where he leads the development, coordination, and implementation of medical policy programs and strategic initiatives. Dr. ElZarrad currently leads multiple projects focused on exploring the potential use of real-world evidence, innovative clinical trial designs, and the integration of technological advances in pharmaceutical development. Dr. ElZarrad is the rapporteur for the International Council for Harmonisation's ongoing work to revise the international Good Clinical Practice Guideline (ICH-E6(R2)). Prior to joining FDA, he served as the acting director of the Clinical and Healthcare Research Policy Division with the Office of Science Policy at the National Institutes of Health (NIH). At NIH, he worked on policies related to human subject protections; the design, conduct, and oversight of clinical research; and the enhancement of quality assurance programs at pharmaceutical development and production facilities. He earned a doctoral degree in medical sciences with a focus on cancer metastases from the University of South Alabama and an M.P.H. from the Johns Hopkins Bloomberg School of Public Health.

Steven K. Galson, M.D., M.P.H., retired from Amgen Inc. in July 2021 nearly 12 years in senior research and development roles as the senior vice president of global regulatory affairs and safety. He joined Amgen in 2010 as the vice president of global regulatory affairs. Prior to Amgen, Dr. Galson was the senior vice president for civilian health operations and the chief health scientist at the Science Applications International Corporation. Dr. Galson spent more than 20 years in government service, including 2 years as acting Surgeon General of the United States. Previously, he served as the director of the U.S. Food and Drug Administration's (FDA's) Center for Drug Evaluation and Research, where he provided leadership for the center's broad national and international programs in pharmaceutical regulation. Dr. Galson began his U.S. Public Health Service (PHS) career as an epidemiological investigator at the Centers for Disease Control and Prevention after completing a residency in internal medicine at the Hospitals of the Medical College of Pennsylvania. He also held senior-level positions at the U.S. Environmental Protection Agency (EPA); the U.S. Department of Energy, where he was the chief medical officer; and the U.S. Department of Health and Human Services. Prior to his arrival at FDA, Dr. Galson was the director of EPA's Office of Science Coordination and Policy, Office of Prevention, Pesticides and Toxic Substances. Dr. Galson holds a B.S. from Stony Brook University, an M.D. from the Icahn School of Medicine at Mount Sinai, and an M.P.H. from the Harvard T.H. Chan School of Public Health. In 2008, he received an honorary doctor of public service degree from the Drexel University School of Public Health, and, in 2015, he received the Jacobi Medallion Award from the Icahn School of Medicine at Mount Sinai. In 2018, Dr. Galson was named the Health Leader of the Year from the Commissioned Officers Association of PHS. Dr. Galson is a member of the Clinical Trials Transformation Initiative Executive Committee and on the Board of Trustees for the Keck Graduate Institute in Claremont, California.

Jennifer Goldsack, M.A., M.B.A., is the executive director at the Digital Medicine Society, a new professional organization promoting the adoption of digital technologies for health. Previously, Ms. Goldsack spent several years at the Clinical Trials Transformation Initiative (CTTI), where she led development and implementation of several projects within CTTI's Mobile Program and was the operational co-lead on the first randomized clinical trial using the U.S. Food and Drug Administration's Sentinel System. Ms. Goldsack spent 5 years working in research at the Hospital of the University of Pennsylvania, first in outcomes research in the Department of Surgery and later in the Department of Medicine. More recently, she helped launch the Value Institute, a pragmatic research and innovation center embedded in a large academic medical center in Delaware. Ms. Goldsack earned her master's degree in chemistry from the University of Oxford, England; her master's degree in history and sociology of medicine from the University of Pennsylvania; and her M.B.A. from The George Washington University. Additionally, she is a Certified Professional in Healthcare Quality.

Tara Hastings, M.A., is the senior associate director of patient engagement at The Michael J. Fox Foundation for Parkinson's Research (MJFF). Ms. Hastings works with both the Parkinson's disease community and key stakeholders across the research and drug therapeutic landscape to ensure the patient perspective is present. She guides MJFF's efforts to foster collaboration and provide guidance on how to meaningfully capture and include patient insights, experiences, desires, and preferences at all phases of development, through mechanisms such as innovative technology platforms, precompetitive consortia, and education initiatives. Ms. Hastings holds a B.A. from Columbia University and an M.A. from the University of Virginia.

Bradford Hirsch, M.D., M.B.A., is the co-founder and the chief executive officer of SignalPath Research, a company leveraging technology to make clinical trials more efficient, effective, and available. He is also a medical oncologist and a principal investigator. Prior to his current focus, he held leadership roles in technology companies and academics, including Flatiron Health and the Duke University School of Medicine. Across all of his roles, he has focused on the use of data and novel technologies to advance the frontier in medicine.

He received his B.A. from the University of Pennsylvania, M.D. from the University of Texas Southwestern, and completed his fellowship and M.B.A. at Duke University. From a clinical perspective, he focuses on treatment and research of genitourinary cancers. He has more than 50 publications in the peer-reviewed literature, continues to speak regularly on topics of medicine and technology, and serves on the American Society of Clinical Oncology cancer research committee, the *Journal of Cancer Clinical Cancer Informatics* editorial board, the National Quality Forum cancer committee, the Parkland Hospital Foundation Board of Directors, and the National Outdoor Leadership School Advisory Board.

Terris King, Sc.D., D.D., M.S., is the senior pastor of Liberty Grace Church of God, the executive director of the Grace Foundation, and a retired federal government senior executive. He is a second-generation ordained Baptist preacher of a growing and vibrant ministry.

Dr. King is the former director and the client executive at AT&T. He was the lead executive for all AT&T services within the U.S. Department of Health and Human Services. These services exceeded $50 million. He previously served as the deputy director of the Office of Information Systems at the Centers for Medicare & Medicaid Services (CMS). The innovation initiatives Dr. King is establishing are CMS's future payment and health care coordination models. Prior this role, Dr. King was the founder of the Office of Minority Health for CMS. In this role, he focused on the establishment of the new office with the mission to improve the health of racial and ethnic minority populations. For 6 years, Dr. King served as the deputy director of the Office of Clinical Standards and Quality (OCSQ), a division of the U.S. Department of Health and Human Services.

Dr. King is a proud alumnus of Walbrook Senior High School in Baltimore, Maryland, from which he graduated and received a scholarship in football. He completed both his scientific doctorate in occupational science and his undergraduate degree in mass communications from Towson University. He completed his master's in behavioral science from Johns Hopkins University and was a Harvard University executive fellow. He received his doctorate in divinity from Saint Thomas College.

Esther Krofah, M.P.P., is the executive director of FasterCures, a center of the Milken Institute. She has deep experience in the government, nonprofit, and for-profit sectors, where she has led efforts to bring together diverse stakeholder groups to solve critical issues and achieve shared goals that improve the lives of patients. Most recently, Ms. Krofah was the director of public policy leading GlaxoSmithKline's (GSK's) engagement with the U.S. Department of Health and Human Services (HHS) and relevant Executive Branch agencies on broad health care policy issues, including leadership in improving vaccinations and care for people living with HIV. Prior to GSK, Ms. Krofah served as the deputy director of HHS's Office of Health Reform, where she led the development of policy positions for significant regulator priorities, including the health insurance marketplaces. Prior to HHS, she served as a program director at the National Governors Association (NGA) health care division, working directly with governors' health policy advisors, state Medicaid directors, and state health commissioners on health insurance, health workforce, and Medicaid coverage issues. Before joining NGA, Ms. Krofah worked in consulting at Deloitte Consulting, LLP, where she worked with public-sector and commercial clients, including assisting states in developing state-based exchanges. Ms. Krofah earned a B.A. from Duke University and an M.P.P. from the Harvard University John F. Kennedy School of Government.

Martin Landray, M.B.Ch.B., Ph.D., FRCP, FHEA, FASN, FBPHS, FESC, is a professor of medicine and epidemiology in the Nuffield Department of Population Health and the deputy director of Oxford's Big Data Institute in the Li Ka Shing Centre for Health Information and Discovery at the University of Oxford. He is a research director for Health Data Research U.K., leading the national program on digitally enabled clinical trials. He leads the Good Clinical Trials Collaborative established by the Wellcome Trust, the Bill & Melinda Gates Foundation, and the African Academy of Sciences. His research seeks to further understand the determinants of common life-threatening and disabling diseases through the design, conduct, and analysis of efficient, large-scale epidemiological studies (including clinical trials) and the widespread dissemination of both the results and the scientific methods used to generate them. The results of his previous trials of treatments for cardiovascular and kidney disease have changed regulatory drug approvals, influenced clinical guidelines, and changed prescribing practice to the benefit of patients. His work on Big Data focuses on the large-scale analysis and interpretation of clinical phenotype through analysis of routine health care data, participant-oriented devices (e.g., smartphones, sensors) and imaging.

Since March 2020, Dr. Landray has been the co-chief investigator of the RECOVERY trial, the national priority platform trial of potential treatments for patients hospitalized with COVID-19 in the United Kingdom. The trial was established at a fast pace, moving from first draft protocol to first patient enrolled in 9 days and randomizing more than 12,000 patients in the first few months. Within the first 100 days, the trial produced three practice-changing results: neither hydroxychloroquine nor lopinavir–ritonavir improve clinical outcomes for hospitalized patients with COVID-19; by contrast, dexamethasone reduces mortality by about one-third for patients requiring invasive mechanical ventilation and by one-fifth for those requiring oxygen. The trial has now enrolled more than 39,000 patients, providing clear evidence that the immunomodulatory drug, tocilizumab, further reduces mortality (and that convalescent plasma, colchicine, and azithromycin do not). The protocol is deliberately streamlined, making extensive use of routine health care data to minimize the burden on clinicians and patients in the context of the ongoing pandemic.

Dr. Landray completed his medical training at University of Birmingham (United Kingdom) and specialist training in clinical pharmacology and therapeutics, and general internal medicine at the University of Birmingham. He continues to practice clinical medicine as an honorary consultant physician in the Department of Cardiology at Oxford University Hospitals National Health Service Trust.

Elliott Levy, M.D., is the senior vice president of research and development (R&D) strategy and operations at Amgen Inc., where he is responsible for delivering the operational and transformational capabilities essential to executing Amgen's R&D strategy. Dr. Levy joined Amgen in 2014 and was the senior vice president of global development, responsible for the clinical development of Amgen's pipeline.

Before joining Amgen, Dr. Levy served as the senior vice president and the head of specialty development at Bristol Myers Squibb (BMS). Prior to that role, he held the position of the senior vice president of global pharmacovigilance and epidemiology. Dr. Levy joined BMS in 1997, and during his 17 years at the company he held a range of senior positions in cardiovascular clinical development, immunoscience clinical research, and global clinical research operations.

Prior to BMS, Dr. Levy was a member of the Renal Division at Brigham and Women's Hospital in Boston, where he was an investigator in federally sponsored outcomes research as well as industry-sponsored clinical trials. Dr. Levy is a graduate of the Yale School of Medicine, where he was chief medical resident and trained in internal medicine and nephrology. He completed fellowship training in clinical research through the Robert Wood Johnson Foundation Clinical Scholars Program at Yale University.

Freda Lewis-Hall, M.D., DFAPA, MFPM, has been on the frontlines of health care as a clinician, educator, researcher, and leader in the biopharmaceuticals and life sciences industries during her 35-year career in medicine. She served as Pfizer Inc.'s chief medical officer and executive vice president until the end of 2018 and as the chief patient officer and the executive vice president during 2019.

Before joining Pfizer, Dr. Lewis-Hall held senior leadership positions of the chief medical officer and the executive vice president, Medicines Development at Vertex Pharmaceuticals; the senior vice president, U.S. Pharmaceuticals at Bristol Myers Squibb; the vice president, research and development, product development at Pharmacia Corporation; and the product team leader and the director at Eli Lilly and Company. Dr. Lewis-Hall currently serves on the Board of Fellows of Harvard Medical School, the Board of Advisors of the Dell Medical School, and the Board of Governors for the Patient-Centered Outcomes Research Institute. She also serves on the corporate boards of Milliken and Company, a global diversified industrial manufacturer; 1Life Healthcare, Inc., a health services company; Exact Sciences, Inc., a molecular diagnostics company; and SpringWorks Therapeutics, a biopharmaceutical company.

Prior to joining the biopharmaceutical industry, Dr. Lewis-Hall served as the vice chair and an associate professor in the Department of Psychiatry at the Howard University College of Medicine and was an advisor to the National Institute of Mental Health. She earned a B.A. in natural sciences from Johns Hopkins University and an M.D. from the Howard University College of Medicine. She launched her medical career as a practicing physician and then focused her academic research on the effects of health care disparities and the impact of mental illness on families and communities.

Dr. Lewis-Hall is a distinguished fellow of the American Psychiatric Association and the Faculty of Pharmaceutical Medicine of the Royal College of Physicians of the United Kingdom. She is a frequent speaker on issues such as improving patient safety and health outcomes, reducing stigma and health care disparities, women's health, public health, corporate leadership, and diversity. Dr. Lewis-Hall is an accomplished developer of consumer education and medical outreach programs, including national television and radio shows such as segments on *Dr. Phil*, *The Doctors*, *The Real*, TEDMed, The Urban Health Report, and multiple online sites.

Mark McClellan, M.D., Ph.D., is the Robert J. Margolis Professor of Business, Medicine, and Policy, and the founding director of the Duke–Margolis Center for Health Policy at Duke University. With offices in Durham, North Carolina, and Washington, DC, the center is a universitywide Duke initiative that is nationally and internationally recognized for research, evaluation, implementation, and educational initiatives to improve health policy and health, most recently in its COVID-19 response. The center integrates Duke's expertise in the social, clinical, and analytical sciences alongside engagement with health care leaders and stakeholders, to develop and apply policy solutions that improve health, health equity, and the value of health care locally, nationally, and worldwide.

Dr. McClellan is a doctor and an economist who has addressed a wide range of strategies and policy reforms to improve health care, including payment reform to promote better outcomes and lower costs, methods for development and use of real-world evidence, and strategies for more effective biomedical innovation.

At the center of the nation's efforts to combat the pandemic, Dr. McClellan is the co-author of a roadmap that details the steps needed for a comprehensive COVID-19 response and safe reopening of our country. His current work on responding to the COVID-19 public health emergency spans virus containment and testing strategies, reforming health care toward more resilient models of delivering care, and accelerating the development of therapeutics and vaccines.

Before coming to Duke, he served as a senior fellow in economic studies at the Brookings Institution, where he was the director of the Health Care Innovation and Value Initiatives and led the Richard Merkin Initiative on Payment Reform and Clinical Leadership. He also has a highly distinguished record in public service and academic research.

Dr. McClellan is a former administrator of the Centers for Medicare & Medicaid Services and the former commissioner of the U.S. Food and Drug Administration (FDA), where he developed and implemented major reforms in health policy. These include the Medicare prescription drug benefit, Medicare and Medicaid payment reforms, FDA's Critical Path Initiative, and public–private initiatives to develop better information on the quality and cost of care. He has also previously served as a member of the President's Council of Economic Advisers and the senior director for health care policy at the White House, and as the deputy assistant secretary for economic policy at the U.S. Department of the Treasury.

Dr. McClellan is the founding chair and a senior advisor of the Reagan–Udall Foundation for FDA, serves on the Institute for Clinical and Economic Review Advisory Board, and is a member of the National Academy of Medicine (NAM). He chairs the NAM's Leadership Council for Value and Science-Driven Health Care, co-chairs the Guiding Committee of the Health Care Payment Learning and Action Network, and is a research associate at the National Bureau of Economic Research. He is also a senior advisor on the faculty of the University of Texas Dell Medical School and an independent director on the boards of Johnson &

Johnson, Cigna, Alignment Healthcare, and PrognomIQ. He was previously an associate professor of economics and medicine with tenure at Stanford University, and has twice received the Kenneth Arrow Award for Outstanding Research in Health Economics.

Marilyn A. Metcalf, Ph.D., leads GlaxoSmithKline's (GSK's) Oncology Patient Council, involving patients in the work of GSK's largest and fastest-growing therapy area. Together they enhance the development and use of innovative treatments and promote understanding of these medicines. As a member of GSK's Global Safety Board, she provides oversight of the safety and benefit–risk balance of GSK's pharma portfolio from First Time in Human through Lifecycle Management. She is a lead author for Council for International Organizations of Medical Sciences (CIOMS) Working Group XI's guidance on patient involvement in the development and safe use of medicines, co-chaired U.S. Patients as Partners 2020, and co-chaired the National Academies of Sciences, Engineering, and Medicine's Science of Patient Input Action Collaborative.

Previously Dr. Metcalf was Family Health International's project director of the National Institutes of Health's master contract for HIV vaccine research focusing on the United States and lower- and middle-income countries. At the former GlaxoWellcome, she studied the safety and efficacy, health economics, and quality of life effects of HIV, oncology, and respiratory therapies. In 2001, she moved with her family to the United Kingdom to rebuild GSK's international Decision Sciences team. After returning to the United States in 2003, she went to Centocor to lead its Decision Sciences and R&D Portfolio Management team. She returned to GSK in 2006 and formed the Benefit–Risk Evaluation team, then led GSK's Pharmacovigilance Centre of Innovation. She began her current role in 2017.

Richard A. Moscicki, M.D., is the executive vice president of science and regulatory advocacy and the chief medical officer at the Pharmaceutical Research and Manufacturers of America (PhRMA). Dr. Moscicki came to PhRMA in 2017 after serving as the deputy center director for science operations for the U.S. Food and Drug Administration's (FDA's) Center for Drug Evaluation and Research (CDER) since 2013. While at FDA, Dr. Moscicki brought executive direction of center operations and leadership in overseeing the development, implementation, and direction of CDER's programs. Previous positions include serving as the chief medical officer at Genzyme Corporation from 1992 to 2011, where he was responsible for worldwide global regulatory and pharmacovigilance matters, as well as all aspects of clinical research and medical affairs for the company. He served as a senior vice president and the head of clinical development at Sanofi-Genzyme from 2011 to 2013.

Dr. Moscicki received his M.D. from the Northwestern University Feinberg Medical School. He is board certified in internal medicine, diagnostic and laboratory immunology, and allergy and immunology. He completed his residency in internal medicine, followed by a fellowship at Massachusetts General Hospital (MGH) in clinical immunology and immunopathology. He remained on staff at MGH and on the faculty of Harvard Medical School from 1979 until 2013.

Megan O'Boyle, B.S., is the parent of a 20-year-old daughter with Phelan-McDermid Syndrome (PMS). She is also the principal investigator for the PMS Data Network (PMS_DN, PCORnet) and the PMS International Registry and the patient engagement lead at RARE-X, a collaborative platform for global data sharing and analysis in rare disease. She advocates for data sharing, collaborating with other advocacy groups, sharing resources, and streamlining institutional review board practices and policies. As the patient engagement lead, she brings her decade of experience in advocacy to help patient groups develop and govern their new data collection efforts within RARE-X. Ms. O'Boyle knows firsthand about the challenges that patients and patient communities face collecting and sharing their data. She is passionate about the need for the rare disease community as a whole to collect standardized data (ask the same questions) to allow for cross-disease research. She believes that having data collection developed and maintained at no cost to the patients and patient communities is imperative to removing the barriers to finding treatments and cures for rare disease. Keeping the patient at the center of all decisions and efforts of RARE-X is Ms. O'Boyle's priority and mission. She serves as a patient advisor on the National Institutes of Health's Council of Councils and the Simons Foundation–SPARK project, is a former advisor to the National Center for Advancing Translational Sciences Advisory Council, and has won several awards, including from FasterCures and Academy Health.

Anaeze Chidiebele Offodile II, M.D., M.P.H., is the executive director for clinical transformation and an assistant professor in the Department of Plastic Surgery at the MD Anderson Cancer Center. Collaborating with key clinical and operational leaders throughout the institution, he is helping to define, align, and implement a high-level roadmap for clinical and economic transformation in support of MD Anderson's vision to deliver high-value cancer care. He is also a non-resident scholar in domestic health policy at the Baker Institute, a non-partisan think tank on the campus of Rice University. His scholarship is focused on examining the subjective and material impacts of patient-borne treatment-related costs ("financial toxicity") and the interaction between vertical integration and the delivery of high-value care. He has received several national awards for his research as well as competitive funding from the Doris Duke Charitable Foundation, the University Cancer Foundation, and the Blue Cross Blue Shield Affordability Cures Consortium. He is currently the 2019–2021 Gilbert Omenn Fellow at the National Academy of Medicine.

A graduate of the Columbia University College of Physicians and Surgeons, he completed surgical training at Brigham & Women's Hospital (general surgery), the Lahey Clinic (Plastic Surgery), and the MD Anderson Cancer Center (microvascular fellowship). Dr. Offodile also received an M.P.H. in health policy from the Johns Hopkins Bloomberg School of Public Health. He previously served as a senior advisor to the director of the Patient Care Models Group (Christina Ritter) at the Center for Medicare & Medicaid Innovation.

Elizabeth Ofili, M.D., M.P.H., FACC, is a professor of medicine at the Morehouse School of Medicine and a practicing cardiologist with Morehouse Healthcare in Atlanta. She serves as the chief medical officer of the Morehouse Choice Accountable Care Organization, a Centers for Medicare & Medicaid Services' Shared Savings Program.

She is a nationally and internationally recognized clinician scientist with particular focus on cardiovascular disparities and women's health. The National Institutes of Health (NIH), as well as industry and foundations, have continuously funded her work since 1994; she has a track record in clinical trials that impact health disparities. In 2002, as the president of the Association of Black Cardiologists, she led the initiative to implement the landmark African American Heart Failure Trial, whose findings led to a change in practice guidelines for the treatment of heart failure in African Americans. She leads or co-leads multi-institutional and national networks funded by NIH to address health disparities and diversity in the biomedical workforce, including the National Research Mentoring Network, an NIH Diversity Program Consortium. She has led collaborative efforts to establish and grow the clinical research infrastructure and training programs at the Morehouse School of Medicine with awards totaling more than $175 million. She has a track record of facilitating cross-institutional research collaborations and community partnerships. These activities include acting as multiple principal investigator (PI) of the Georgia Clinical and Translational Science Alliance, the statewide collaboration at Emory University, the Morehouse School of Medicine, the Georgia Institute of Technology, and the University of Georgia, and partnering with health systems and statewide research organizations totaling more than 1,558 investigators, 49 scholars, 112 trainees, and 110 other career development students. She serves as contact PI for the Research Centers at Minority Institutions (RCMI) Coordinating

Center, which works with all 21 National Institute on Minority Health and Health Disparities–funded RCMI U54 Centers at Historically Black, Hispanic/Minority Serving, and Native Hawaiian/Pacific Islander Serving Institutions to support investigator development, and data standards for evaluation across the consortium. She was lead author of a publication on models of partnerships between Historically Black Colleges and Universities/Minority Serving Institutions (HBCUs/MSIs) and research-intensive institutions.

Dr. Ofili has delivered more than 700 scientific presentations and published more than 150 scientific papers in national and international journals. As the American Association of Medical Colleges 2007 Council of Dean Fellow, Dr. Ofili led a project on best practices to sustaining the biomedical and physician workforce.

Dr. Ofili brings her knowledge of health and medicine to technology and innovation. She is the founder and the chief science officer of AccuHealth Technologies Inc. (www.Myaccuhealth.com) and Health 360x, a patient engagement and health coaching platform that empowers patients in their journey from health care to wellness. Health 360x platform is testing innovative approaches to integrate real-world data from electronic medical records to support research participation by patients and providers that are underrepresented in clinical trials. Dr. Ofili holds a patent for "A system and method for chronic illness care," and has received more than 50 national awards, including "Changing the Face of Medicine: The Rise of America's Women Physicians" Exhibit at the National Library of Medicine. She is an elected member of the National Academy of Medicine (2015). She is an elected member of the Association of University Cardiologists (2007) and the American Clinical and Climatological Association (2016). She has advised NIH on diversity in the biomedical research workforce, and served on the board of directors of the National Space Biomedical Research Institute. Dr. Ofili currently serves as the chair of the Board of Directors of the Association of Black Cardiologists, whose motto is "Saving the Hearts and Minds of a Diverse America" (www.abcardio.org).

Amy Patterson, M.D., is the chief science advisor and the director of scientific research programs, policy, and strategic initiatives in the Immediate Office of the Director of the National Heart, Lung, and Blood Institute (NHLBI), part of the National Institutes of Health (NIH). In this role, she provides leadership and strategic coordination of trans-NHLBI efforts and manages a broad portfolio of issues germane to the conduct of clinical research, research oversight, policy development, major new scientific initiatives, and relationships with organizations within and external to the Institute.

Prior to joining NHLBI in 2015, Dr. Patterson served as the NIH associate director for science policy and as the NIH associate director for biosecurity and biosafety policy. Her responsibilities encompassed areas such as human subjects protections; the organization and oversight of clinical trials; scientific, social, and ethical considerations in genetics research and human gene transfer trials; and safety and security implications of emerging new technologies.

Prior to coming to NIH's Office of the Director, she served as the deputy director of the Division of Cellular and Gene Therapies and the medical officer in the Division of Clinical Trial Design and Analysis at the U.S. Food and Drug Administration's Center for Biologics Evaluation and Research. Dr. Patterson received her B.A. (cum laude) in biology from Harvard University and her M.D. (Alpha Omega Alpha) from the Albert Einstein College of Medicine. She conducted her internship and residency in internal medicine at New York Hospital and Memorial Sloan Kettering and completed her postdoctoral clinical research fellowships in adult and pediatric endocrinology and metabolism at NIH.

Eric Perakslis, Ph.D., is the chief science and digital officer at the Duke Clinical Research Institute. He was previously a Rubenstein Fellow at Duke University, where his work focused on collaborative efforts in data science that spanned medicine, policy, engineering, computer science, information technology, and security. Immediately prior to his arrival at Duke, Dr. Perakslis served as the chief scientific advisor at Datavant, a lecturer in the Department of Biomedical Informatics at Harvard Medical School, and a strategic innovation advisor to the Médecins Sans Frontières.

Dr. Perakslis was the senior vice president and the head of the Takeda R&D Data Science Institute, where he built an integrated institute of more than 165 multidisciplinary data scientists serving all aspects of biopharmaceutical research and development (R&D) and digital health. Prior to Takeda, Dr. Perakslis was the executive director of the Center for Biomedical Informatics and the Countway Library of Medicine, an instructor in pediatrics at Harvard Medical School (HMS), and a faculty member of the Children's Hospital Informatics Program at Boston Children's Hospital.

During his time at HMS, Dr. Perakslis focused on the approval of the Department of Biomedical Informatics as a full academic department, the development of the National Institutes of Health's Undiagnosed Diseases Network, industry collaborations, leading the technology efforts for multiple Ebola response programs, and building active research programs in medical product development, regulatory science, and cybersecurity.

Prior to HMS, Dr. Perakslis served as the chief information officer and chief scientist (informatics) at the U.S. Food and Drug Administration

(FDA). In this role, he authored the first information technology (IT) Strategic Plan for FDA and was responsible for modernizing and enhancing the IT capabilities as well as in silico scientific capabilities at FDA.

Prior to his time at FDA, Dr. Perakslis was the senior vice president of R&D information technology at Johnson & Johnson (J&J) Pharmaceuticals R&D and a member of the Corporate Office of Science and Technology. While at J&J, he created and open-sourced the tranSMART clinical data system, which is now being freely used by hundreds of health care organizations. During his 13 years at J&J, he also held the posts of the vice president of R&D informatics, the vice president and the chief information officer, the director of research information technology, and the director of drug discovery research. Prior to working at J&J, Dr. Perakslis was the group leader of scientific computing at ArQule Inc.

Dr. Perakslis has served on the editorial board of *Cancer Today* magazine and as the associate editor for novel communications for the *Journal of Therapeutic Innovation and Regulatory Science*. He has also served on science and technology advisory committees and in leadership roles for the American Society of Clinical Oncology, NuMedii, Precision for Medicine, the Survivor Advisory Board at the Cancer Institute of New Jersey, the Kidney Cancer Association, OneMind4Research, and the Scientist-Survivor program of the American Association for Cancer Research. Internationally, he has served as the chief information officer of the King Hussein Institute for Biotechnology and Cancer in Amman, Jordan. Dr. Perakslis has a Ph.D. in chemical and biochemical engineering from Drexel University. He also holds a B.S.Ch.E. and an M.S. in chemical engineering.

Eliseo Pérez-Stable, M.D., is the director of the National Institutes of Health's (NIH's) National Institute on Minority Health and Health Disparities, which seeks to advance the science of minority health and health disparities research through research, training, research capacity development, public education, and information dissemination. Dr. Pérez-Stable practiced general internal medicine for 37 years at the University of California, San Francisco (UCSF), before moving to NIH in 2015. He was a professor of medicine at UCSF and the chief of the Division of General Internal Medicine for 17 years. His research interests include improving the health of racial and ethnic minorities and underserved populations, advancing patient-centered care, improving cross-cultural communication skills among clinicians, and promoting diversity in the biomedical research workforce. For more than 30 years, Dr. Pérez-Stable led research on Latino smoking cessation and tobacco control policy in the United States and Latin America, addressing clinical and prevention issues in cancer screening, and mentoring more than 70 minority investigators. He has published more than 250 peer-reviewed articles and was elected to the National Academy of Medicine in 2001.

Sam Roosz, M.B.A., is the chief executive officer and the co-founder of Crescendo Health, a health care technology company that supports trial sponsors in integrating real-world evidence into their study designs. Mr. Roosz previously co-founded Datavant, the leading vendor of privacy preserving record linkage, where he served as the general manager of life sciences. Mr. Roosz previously held roles at Natera, Element Science, and Putnam Associates. He holds a degree in molecular and cellular biology from Harvard University and an M.B.A. from Stanford University.

Bárbara Segarra-Vázquez, D.H.Sc., has been a faculty member at the University of Puerto Rico for 30 years. She is the dean of the School of Health Professions and one of the principal investigators of the Hispanic Clinical and Translational Research Education and Career Development program (R25MD007607) funded by the National Institutes of Health. Dr. Segarra-Vázquez was diagnosed with breast cancer Stage IIB on 2003 and was in remission for 13 years. In 2017, she had a recurrence of metastatic breast cancer to the skin. A volunteer for Komen Puerto Rico since 2006, she was the board president for 4 years. She is a member of the Puerto Rico Cancer Control Coalition, currently serving as the leader of the survivorship committee. She has served several times as a consumer reviewer for the Breast Cancer Research Program of the U.S. Department of Defense's Congressionally Directed Medical Research Programs and traveled to Komen Global Initiative to meet with different groups that provided services to breast cancer patients and participate in a public activity of breast cancer awareness. She is the vice chair of the Steering Committee for Komen Advocates in Science and a member of the Southwest Oncology Group Cancer Research Network Patient Advocates Committee. She is the founder and the co-investigator of Hispanics Increasing Diversity to Enhance Advocacy in Science.

Brian Southwell, Ph.D., is the senior director of the Science in the Public Sphere Program in RTI International's Center for Communication Science. He also is an adjunct professor and Duke–RTI Scholar with Duke University and a graduate faculty member and an adjunct associate professor at the University of North Carolina at Chapel Hill. In more than 100 articles, chapters, and books, including *Misinformation and Mass Audiences* and *Social Networks and Popular Understanding of Science and Health*, Dr. Southwell has explored public understanding of science. At Duke, he has been involved with a series of year-long faculty–student projects on topics such as residential energy use behavior and public engagement regarding air pollution. Dr. Southwell hosts WNCU's *The Measure of Everyday Life*, speaks at events such as the Aspen Ideas Festival, and advises for NOVA *Science Studio*.

Pamela Tenaerts, M.D., M.B.A., is the chief scientific officer at Medable, where she directs research to help identify, implement, and make ubiquitous responsible decentralized trial strategies. Dr. Tenaerts brings more than 30 years of experience in clinical trials, as a researcher and academic, in medical device research operations, as a hospital-based site administrator, and as a physician, most recently serving as the executive director of the Clinical Trials Transformation Initiative (CTTI), a multistakeholder public–private partnership to improve quality and efficiency in clinical trials at Duke University. She sits on the boards of the Society of Clinical Trials and the Scientific Leadership Council of the Digital Medicine Society, participates in the Good Clinical Trial Collaborative, and is a member of the National Academies of Science, Engineering, and Medicine's Forum on Drug Discovery, Development, and Translation. She received her M.D. from Catholic University in Leuven, Belgium, and her M.B.A. from the University of South Florida.

Jonathan Watanabe, Pharm.D., Ph.D., BCGP, is a professor of clinical pharmacy and an associate director and the founding associate dean of assessment and quality at the University of California, Irvine, Samueli College of Health Sciences and a National Academy of Medicine Emerging Leader in Health and Medicine scholar. He was a contributor to the National Academies of Sciences, Engineering, and Medicine's *Making Medicines Affordable: A National Imperative* consensus study report and is a current member of the National Academies' ad hoc Committee on Implications of Discarded Weight-Based Drugs. Dr. Watanabe employs real-world data to develop policy solutions to improve patient care, augment population health, and reduce medical costs. Dr. Watanabe focuses on improving access to evidence-driven medication use and pharmacist-directed patient care. He serves as an advisor to the California Health Benefits Review Program for the California State Legislature. His research on safe and effective medication use has been cited in enacted legislation efforts. He served as an investigator, faculty, and fellowship director for the federal Health Resources and Services Administration–funded San Diego Geriatrics Workforce Enhancement Program and is a current investigator for the California Tobacco-Related Disease Research Program. Dr. Watanabe was the inaugural recipient of the University of Washington (UW)/Allergan Global Health Economics and Outcomes Research Fellowship. He served as a clinical consultant at the San Diego Program of All-inclusive Care for the Elderly Clinic. He is an advisor to the Joint Commission on pain management and assessment standards in long-term care. He received his B.S. from UW. He received a Pharm.D. from the University of Southern California. He received an M.S. and a Ph.D. from UW's Comparative Health Outcomes, Policy, and Economics Institute. He is a board-certified geriatric pharmacist.

Janet Woodcock, M.D., was named the acting commissioner of food and drugs on January 20, 2021. As the acting commissioner, Dr. Woodcock oversees the full breadth of the U.S. Food and Drug Administration (FDA) portfolio and execution of the Federal Food, Drug, and Cosmetic Act and other applicable laws. This includes ensuring the safety, effectiveness, and security of human and veterinary drugs, vaccines and other biological products for human use, and medical devices; the safety and security of our nation's food supply, cosmetics, dietary supplements, and products that give off electronic radiation; and the regulation of tobacco products.

Dr. Woodcock began her FDA career in 1984, joining the Center for Biologics Evaluation and Research (CBER) as the director of the Division of Biological Investigational New Drugs, as well as serving as CBER's acting deputy director for a period of time. She later became the director of the Office of Therapeutics Research and Review in CBER, which included the approval of the first biotechnology-based treatments for multiple sclerosis and cystic fibrosis during her tenure.

In 1994, Dr. Woodcock was named the director of FDA's Center for Drug Evaluation and Research (CDER), overseeing the center's work that is the world's gold standard for drug approval and safety. There she led many of FDA's drug initiatives, including introducing the concept of risk management as a new approach to drug safety; modernizing drug manufacturing and regulation through the Pharmaceutical Quality for the 21st Century Initiative; advancing medical discoveries from the laboratory to consumers more efficiently under the Critical Path Initiative; and launching the Safety First and Safe Use initiatives designed to improve drug safety management within and outside FDA, respectively.

In 2004, Dr. Woodcock became the deputy commissioner and the chief medical officer in the Office of the Commissioner. Later she took on other executive leadership positions in the Commissioner's Office, including the deputy commissioner for operations and the chief operating officer.

In 2007, Dr. Woodcock returned as the director of CDER until she was asked to lend her expertise to Operation Warp Speed for developing therapeutics during the COVID-19 pandemic, such as evaluating the potential benefits of monoclonal antibody treatments for certain COVID-19 patients. From late 2020, she split her time advising Operation Warp Speed on advancing COVID-19 therapeutics with serving as the principal medical advisor to the commissioner on key priorities on behalf of the Office of the Commissioner.

Dr. Woodcock holds a B.S. in chemistry from Bucknell University and an M.D. from the Northwestern University Feinberg School of Medicine. She also completed further training and a fellowship in rheumatology and held teaching appointments at The Pennsylvania State University and the University of California, San Francisco. She is board certified in internal medicine. Dr. Woodcock has been bestowed numerous honors over her distinguished public health career, most notably: a Lifetime Achievement Award in 2015 from the Institute for Safe Medication Practices; the Ellen V. Sigal Advocacy Leadership Award in 2016 from Friends of Cancer Research; the Florence Kelley Consumer Leadership Award in 2017 from the National Consumers League; and the 2019 Biotechnology Heritage Award from the Biotechnology Innovation Organization and Science History Institute.

Appendix C

Workshop Agendas

**Envisioning a Transformed Clinical Trials Enterprise for 2030:
A Virtual Workshop
January 26, February 9, March 24, and May 11, 2021**

> This virtual public workshop will provide a venue for stakeholders to consider a transformed clinical trials enterprise for 2030. Workshop participants will consider lessons learned from progress and setbacks over the past 10 years, since the previous workshop, Envisioning a Transformed Clinical Trials Enterprise in the United States, and, looking forward, discuss goals and key priorities for advancing a clinical trials enterprise that is more efficient, effective, person-centered, inclusive, and integrated into the health delivery system of 2030.
> This virtual workshop was conducted in four parts:
>
> - Part One (January 26, 2021) provided an overview discussion on how an envisioned 2030 clinical trials enterprise may differ from the current system. It discussed key challenges and opportunities in improving person-centeredness and inclusivity, building resilience and transparency, and integrating new technologies.
> - Part Two (February 9, 2021) considered achievable goals to enhance person-centeredness and inclusivity in the clinical trials enterprise and discussed ways to improve public engagement and partnership.
> - Part Three (March 24, 2021) considered approaches to building resilience, sustainability, and transparency. The discussion included the convergence and integration of clinical research and clinical practice; data sharing and management; and efficient, engaging scientific communication.

- Part Four (May 11, 2021) considered ways the thoughtful and deliberate use of new technologies could improve the clinical trials enterprise and support goals outlined in prior webinar sessions.

For additional information on the virtual workshop, please visit the main project page at https://www.nationalacademies.org/our-work/envisioning-a-transformed-clinical-trials-enterprise-for-2030-a-workshop.

Workshop Part 1: January 26, 2021
11:00 a.m.–3:30 p.m. ET

11:00 a.m. **Welcome and Opening Remarks**
STEVEN GALSON, *Workshop Co-Chair*
Senior Vice President, Global Regulatory Affairs and Safety
Amgen Inc.

ESTHER KROFAH, *Workshop Co-Chair*
Executive Director
FasterCures, Milken Institute

SESSION I
A MORE PERSON-CENTERED AND INCLUSIVE CLINICAL TRIALS ENTERPRISE

Session Objective:
- Discuss key priority challenges and opportunities when it comes to person-centeredness and inclusivity in the 2030 clinical trials enterprise

11:10 a.m. **A Story in Action: Person-Centeredness and Inclusivity**
TERRIS KING
Former Director, Office of Minority Health
Centers for Medicare & Medicaid Services

11:25 a.m. **Facilitated Breakout Groups** *(30 min)*

Discussion Questions:
- *Do you agree with the proposed goals listed below for enhancing person-centeredness and inclusivity?*
- *What would you change, and how?*
- *What are potential interim actions or milestones that might be key to achieving these goals?*

Goals to Consider for Enhancing Person-Centeredness and Inclusivity
- Improve representation and relevance
- Improve community engagement, transparency, and "user-friendliness" to foster trust, counter misinformation, and meet the needs of patients
- Demonstrate trustworthiness to the general public of clinical trials
- Engage and prepare a diverse clinical research workforce

11:55 a.m. **Breakout Group Report-Outs** *(10 min)*

12:10 p.m. **BREAK** *(30 min)*

SESSION II
A MORE RESILIENT, SUSTAINABLE, AND TRANSPARENT CLINICAL TRIALS ENTERPRISE

Session Objective:
- Discuss key priority challenges and opportunities when it comes to building a more resilient, sustainable, and transparent clinical trials enterprise

12:45 p.m. **The State of Clinical Trials in 2021: A Perspective from Industry**
ELLIOTT LEVY
Senior Vice President, R&D Strategy and Operations
Amgen Inc.

1:00 p.m. **A Story in Action: Building a More Resilient, Sustainable, and Transparent Clinical Trials Enterprise**
JANET WOODCOCK
Acting Commissioner of Food and Drugs
U.S. Food and Drug Administration

1:15 p.m.   **Facilitated Breakout Groups** *(30 min)*

Discussion Questions:
- *Do you agree with the straw vision statement for building a more resilient, sustainable, and transparent clinical trials enterprise (below)?*
- *What would you change, and how?*
- *What are some potential interim actions or milestones that might be key to achieving these goals?*

Goals to Consider for Building a More Resilient, Sustainable, and Transparent Clinical Trials Enterprise
- Improve community engagement, transparency, and "user-friendliness" to foster trust, counter misinformation, and meet the needs of patients
- Reduce complexity and streamline trials and trial start-up, and standardize key data elements
- Support regulatory robustness, flexibility, and built-in ability to adjust (e.g., in times of stress, to handle new tech robustly)
- Reduce conduction of "uninformative" clinical trials and prioritize resources to robustly designed trials
- Generate a larger amount of high-quality evidence at lower cost
- Reduce risk aversion to improve research questions and trial design innovation
- Embrace novel statistical techniques to power trials
- Connect and embed clinical care and clinical research

1:45 p.m.   **Breakout Group Report-Outs** *(10 min)*

2:00 p.m.   **BREAK** *(30 min)*

SESSION III
MORE APPROPRIATE USE OF TECHNOLOGIES TO OPTIMIZE THE CLINICAL TRIALS ENTERPRISE

Session Objective:
- Discuss key priority challenges and opportunities when it comes to appropriately using new technologies to optimize the 2030 clinical trials enterprise

2:30 p.m. **A Story in Action: Optimizing with New Technologies**
Robert Califf
Head of Clinical Policy and Strategy
Verily Life Sciences and Google Health

2:45 p.m. **Facilitated Breakout Groups** *(30 min)*

Discussion Questions:
- *Do you agree with the proposed goals listed below for more appropriately using new technologies to optimize the clinical trials enterprise?*
- *What would you change, and how?*
- *What are some potential interim actions or milestones that might be key to achieving these goals?*

Goals to Consider for More Appropriately Using Technology to Optimize the Clinical Trials Enterprise
- Decentralize clinical trials
- Use digital tools for clinical trials management
- Develop resources to help institutions that need more support
- Increase local capacity for research innovation
- Collate efforts to frame new technologies as part of an ecosystem rather than a series of unrelated one-off tech solutions
- Develop and deploy systems and tools to combine many sources of data
- Incorporate patient input into research
- Advance analytics for recruitment and analysis

3:15 p.m. **Breakout Group Report-Outs** *(10 min)*

WRAP-UP

3:30 p.m. **Wrap-Up Discussion and Closing Remarks**
Steven Galson, *Workshop Co-Chair*
Senior Vice President, Global Regulatory Affairs and Safety
Amgen Inc.

Esther Krofah, *Workshop Co-Chair*
Executive Director
FasterCures, Milken Institute

3:35 p.m. **ADJOURN**

Workshop Part 2: February 9, 2021
Enhancing Outcomes in a More Person-Centered and Inclusive Clinical Trials Enterprise
11:00 a.m.–3:00 p.m. ET

11:00 a.m. **Welcome and Opening Remarks**
STEVEN GALSON, *Workshop Co-Chair*
Senior Vice President, Research & Development
Amgen Inc.

ESTHER KROFAH, *Workshop Co-Chair*
Executive Director
FasterCures, Milken Institute

LUTHER CLARK, *Moderator*
Deputy Chief Patient Officer and Global Director, Scientific, Medical, and Patient Perspective
Merck & Co., Inc.

SESSION I
THE ROAD TO 2030: AN ATLAS FOR CHANGE

11:10 a.m. **Frontline Experience: A Fireside Chat**
ESTHER KROFAH, *Moderator*
Executive Director
FasterCures, Milken Institute

ELISEO PÉREZ-STABLE
Director
National Institute on Minority Health and Health Disparities
National Institutes of Health

RICHARDAE ARAOJO
Associate Commissioner for Minority Health
Director, Office of Minority Health and Health Equity
U.S. Food and Drug Administration

MEGAN O'BOYLE
Principal Investigator
Phelan-McDermid Syndrome Registry

11:45 a.m. **Charge to the Breakout Groups**

11:50 a.m. **"Lightning Round" Breakout Discussion Groups** *(30 min)*

- *What are one to two short-term, tangible, and measurable goals to ensure a more person-centered and inclusive clinical trials enterprise that should be met within the next 5 years—by 2025?*
- *What technologies, tools, or techniques could be transformational to improving inclusiveness and equity in the clinical trials enterprise over the next 5 years?*

12:30 p.m. **Session I Wrap-Up** *(10 min)*

12:45 p.m. **BREAK** *(30 min)*

SESSION II THE ROAD TO 2030: A CALL TO ACTION

1:15 p.m. **"North-Star" Visions of What Is Possible** *(10 min each)*
Silas Buchanan
Chief Executive Officer
Institute for eHealth Equity

Marilyn A. Metcalf
Senior Director, Patient Engagement
GlaxoSmithKline

1:40 p.m. **Frontline Experience: A Road Already Traveled**
Margaret Anderson
Consulting Managing Director, Strategy and Analytics
Deloitte

1:50 p.m. **Charge to the Breakout Groups**

2:00 p.m. **"Lightning Round" Breakout Discussion Groups** *(30 min)*

- *What are one to two long-term, tangible, and measurable goals to ensure a more person-centered and inclusive clinical trials enterprise that should be met within the next 10 years—by 2030?*
- *What technologies, tools, or techniques could be transformational to improving inclusiveness and equity in the clinical trials enterprise over the next 10 years?*

2:30 p.m. **Session II Wrap-Up** *(10 min)*

WRAP-UP

2:45 p.m. **Wrap-Up Discussion and Closing Remarks**
LUTHER CLARK, *Moderator*
Deputy Chief Patient Officer and Global Director, Scientific, Medical, and Patient Perspective
Merck & Co., Inc.

ESTHER KROFAH, *Workshop Co-Chair*
Executive Director
FasterCures, Milken Institute

STEVEN GALSON, *Workshop Co-Chair*
Senior Vice President, Research & Development
Amgen Inc.

3:00 p.m. **ADJOURN**

Workshop Part 3: March 24, 2021
Building a More Resilient, Sustainable, and Transparent Clinical Trials Enterprise
11:00 a.m.–3:00 p.m. Eastern Time

11:00 a.m. **Welcome and Opening Remarks**
STEVEN GALSON, *Workshop Co-Chair*
Senior Vice President, Research & Development
Amgen Inc.

ESTHER KROFAH, *Workshop Co-Chair*
Executive Director
FasterCures, Milken Institute

SESSION I
THE ROAD TO 2030: AN ATLAS FOR CHANGE

CHRISTOPHER AUSTIN, *Moderator*
Director
National Center for Translational Sciences
National Institutes of Health

11:10 a.m.	**Keynote Address** Martin Landray Professor of Medicine and Epidemiology Nuffield Department of Population Health University of Oxford
11:25 a.m.	**Frontline Experience: A Panel Discussion** *Physician's perspective on a true "Learning Health Care System"* Elizabeth Ofili Contact Principal Investigator Research Centers at Minority Institutions Coordinating Center *Patient's perspective on sustainability* Bárbara Segarra-Vázquez Dean School of Health Professions, Medical Sciences Campus University of Puerto Rico *Industry perspective on building community-based research infrastructure* Freda Lewis-Hall Retired Senior Medical Advisor Pfizer Inc.
12:00 p.m.	**Charge to the Breakout Groups**
12:05 p.m.	**"Lightning Round" Breakout Discussion Groups** *(40 min)* *Discussion Questions:* • What are one to two short-term, tangible, and measurable goals to ensure a more resilient, sustainable, and transparent clinical trials enterprise that should be met within the next 5 years—by 2025? • What technologies, tools, or techniques could be transformational to improving resilience, sustainability, and transparency in the clinical trials enterprise over the next 5 years? • What are specific models of sustainability, resilience, or transparency that participants have encountered in the past year that might be informative for the clinical trials enterprise, and could they be scaled (in part or in whole)?

12:45 p.m. **Breakout Group Wrap-Up**
CHRISTOPHER AUSTIN, *Moderator*
Director
National Center for Translational Sciences
National Institutes of Health

12:55 p.m. **BREAK** *(30 min)*

SESSION II
THE ROAD TO 2030: A CALL TO ACTION

KHAIR ELZARRAD, *Moderator*
Deputy Director
Office of Medical Policy
U.S. Food and Drug Administration

1:30 p.m. **"North-Star" Vision of What Is Possible**
BRIAN SOUTHWELL
Senior Director, Science in the Public Sphere Program
RTI International

1:45 p.m. **Frontline Experience: A Road Already Traveled**
DYAN BRYSON
Founder, Patient Engagement Strategist
Inspired Health Strategies

PAMELA TENAERTS
Former Executive Director
Clinical Trials Transformation Initiative

2:10 p.m. **Charge to the Breakout Groups**

2:15 p.m. **"Lightning Round" Breakout Discussion Groups** *(30 min)*

Discussion Questions:
- What are one to two long-term, tangible, and measurable goals to ensure a more resilient, sustainable, and transparent clinical trials enterprise that should be met within the next 10 years — by 2030?
- What technologies, tools, or techniques could be transformational to improving resilience, sustainability, and transparency in the clinical trials enterprise over the next 10 years?

- *What are specific models of sustainability, resilience, or transparency that participants have encountered in the past year that might be informative for the clinical trials enterprise, and could they be scaled (in part or in whole)?*

2:45 p.m. **Breakout Group Wrap-Up and Closing Remarks**
Khair ElZarrad, *Moderator*
Deputy Director
Office of Medical Policy
U.S. Food and Drug Administration

Steven Galson, *Workshop Co-Chair*
Senior Vice President, Research & Development
Amgen Inc.

Esther Krofah, *Workshop Co-Chair*
Executive Director
FasterCures, Milken Institute

3:00 p.m. **ADJOURN**

Workshop Part 4: May 11, 2021
Practical Applications for Technology to Enhance the Clinical Trials Enterprise
11:00 a.m.–3:00 p.m. ET

11:00 a.m. **Welcome and Opening Remarks**
Steven Galson, *Workshop Co-Chair*
Senior Vice President, Research & Development
Amgen Inc.

Esther Krofah, *Workshop Co-Chair*
Executive Director
FasterCures, Milken Institute

SESSION I
THE ROAD TO 2030: AN ATLAS FOR CHANGE

Jennifer Goldsack, *Moderator*
Executive Director
Digital Medicine Society

11:10 a.m. **Keynote Address**
AMY ABERNETHY
Former Principal Deputy Commissioner of Food and Drugs
U.S. Food and Drug Administration

11:25 a.m. **Frontline Experience: A Panel Discussion**
A perspective on patient burden and accessibility
TARA HASTINGS
Senior Associate Director of Patient Engagement
The Michael J. Fox Foundation for Parkinson's Research

A perspective on digital law
JAN BENEDIKT BRÖNNEKE
Director, Law & Economics Health Technologies
health innovation hub

A perspective on improving software and experience for clinical trial sites
BRADFORD HIRSCH
Chief Executive Officer
SignalPath Research

11:55 a.m. **Charge to the Breakout Groups**

12:00 p.m. **"Lightning Round" Breakout Discussion Groups** *(25 min)*

The breakout groups will be assigned one of the two following goals and asked to discuss practical applications and partnerships with new technologies that can address key priority challenges, and opportunities aligned with this goal that will move us toward the clinical trials enterprise envisioned for 2030. See associated breakout discussion guides for more detail.
- **GOAL 1: Enable a more person-centered and easily accessible clinical trials enterprise.** This also relates to the vision of the Clinical Trials Transformation Initiative for 2030: https://www.ctti-clinicaltrials.org/transforming-trials-2030
- **GOAL 2: Simplify trials (less data collection, fewer site visits) and lower costs while still generating high-quality data and robust answers to relevant research questions.**

12:25 p.m. **Breakout Group Wrap-Up**

FIRESIDE CHAT

12:30 p.m. **Fireside Chat**
Mark McClellan
Director
Duke–Margolis Center for Health Policy

Amy Abernethy, *Moderator*
Former Principal Deputy Commissioner of Food and Drugs
U.S. Food and Drug Administration

1:00 p.m. **BREAK** *(30 min)*

SESSION II
THE ROAD TO 2030: A CALL TO ACTION

Anita Allen, *Moderator*
Henry R. Silverman Professor of Law, Professor of Philosophy
University of Pennsylvania Carey Law School

1:30 p.m. **Frontline Experience: A Road Already Traveled**
Janice Chang
Chief Operating Officer
TransCelerate BioPharma Inc.

Pamela Tenaerts
Chief Scientific Officer
Medable

1:50 p.m. **Charge to the Breakout Groups**

2:00 p.m. **"Lightning Round" Breakout Discussion Groups** *(25 min)*

The breakout groups will be assigned one of the two following goals and asked to discuss practical applications and partnerships with new technologies that can address key priority challenges, and opportunities aligned with this goal that will move us toward the clinical trials enterprise envisioned for 2030.
- **GOAL 3:** Establish a clinical trials enterprise that is diverse, equitable, and inclusive.
- **GOAL 4:** Establish a national network of community-based clinical trial sites.

2:25 p.m. **Breakout Group Wrap-Up**

CLOSING PANEL

2:35 p.m. **A "North-Star" Vision of What Is Possible**
Andy Coravos
Chief Executive Officer and Co-Founder
Elektra Labs

Eric Perakslis
Chief Science and Digital Officer
Duke Clinical Research Institute

Sam Roosz
Co-Founder and Chief Executive Officer
Crescendo Health

2:55 p.m. **Workshop Wrap-Up**
Steven Galson, *Workshop Co-Chair*
Senior Vice President, Research & Development
Amgen Inc.

Esther Krofah, *Workshop Co-Chair*
Executive Director
FasterCures, Milken Institute

3:00 p.m. **ADJOURN**